The Interruption That We Are

Studies in Rhetoric/Communication
Thomas W. Benson, Series Editor

The Interruption That We Are

The Health of the Lived Body, Narrative, and Public Moral Argument

MICHAEL J. HYDE

THE UNIVERSITY OF SOUTH CAROLINA PRESS

Published by the University of South Carolina Press
Columbia, South Carolina 29208

www.sc.edu/uscpress

Manufactured in the United States of America

27 26 25 24 23 22 21 20 19 18
10 9 8 7 6 5 4 3 2 1

Library of Congress Cataloging-in-Publication Data
can be found at http://catalog.loc.gov/.

ISBN: 978-1-61117-707-7 (hardback)
ISBN: 978-1-61117-708-4 (ebook)

This book was printed on recycled paper with 30 percent
postconsumer waste content.

For Dr. Ralph Webb Jr., my M.A and Ph.D. director,
whose support and wisdom were a blessing

Contents

Series Editor's Preface

In *The Interruption That We Are,* Michael J. Hyde confronts the annoyance of being interrupted and turns it on itself to notice that interruption is the condition of our being, mirrored in the interruption that we are, inviting us to see our interrupted and interruptive experience as requiring us to cultivate eloquence in public moral argument.

Professor Hyde shows us how the most mundane, everyday experience of interruption can lead us to a human quest for understanding of how interruption defines our condition as humans—in religion ("In the beginning . . ."), science, philosophy, medical ethics, and rhetoric.

Hyde invokes and critically reads the Judeo-Christian biblical tradition, and the philosophical writings of Søren Kierkegaard, Martin Heidegger, and Emmanuel Levinas, before turning to a series of case studies of public moral argument. A patient suffering from heart disease receives an experimental artificial heart, a case in which scientific medicine, a mechanical device, and a rhetoric of heroic perfection seem to challenge the human narrative of suffering and dignity thus interrupted. Hyde narrates the case of disability rights activist and attorney Harriet McBryde Johnson, who was born with a degenerative neuromuscular disease, and examines her debate with Princeton philosophy professor Peter Singer, whose theories of eugenics would, had they been applied, almost certainly have ended Johnson's life before it began. How could these two beings possibly talk with each other? But they did, and, though neither compromised, Hyde finds in their debate and in Singer's obituary for Johnson an acknowledgment that, in Hyde's estimation, manages to find the right words even without compromising. Brittany Maynard, diagnosed with terminal brain cancer, chose to die by medically assisted suicide, leaving behind a testamentary video describing her choice. The video and the public response when it was placed online constitute a moment of public moral argument between Maynard and Kara Tippetts, who herself later died of cancer without resorting to medically assisted euthanasia. A final chapter scouts our prospects in a posthuman future.

In *The Interruption That We Are,* Michael Hyde displays an experience deeply rooted in day-to-day human existence and in his years of observation and interaction with the practices of medicine and the lives of patients. He develops a conscientious attention to the circumstances and the words of human moral argument about life and death matters, with a scrupulous responsibility to the philosophical tradition, to the claims and virtues of competing arguments, and to the necessity for judgment. Our privilege as readers of *The Interruption That We Are* is to be spectators, students, and beneficiaries of this master teacher.

THOMAS W. BENSON

Preface

It was one of those days. Too many interruptions. I hadn't slept well the night before, waking up numerous times feeling exhausted. My writing was hitting road blocks. I was going to be late for an early morning meeting. I had a minor disagreement with my wife. I couldn't find my car keys. I couldn't find a parking place at the university. I dropped my books and computer on the pavement when I exited the car. When I reached my office I found a voicemail that indicated that I had to attend an emergency research meeting at the medical school after my classes. My undergraduate and graduate seminar did not go as smoothly as I had planned. A meeting with one of my thesis advisees was less than rewarding. By the time I returned home from the medical school, I was exhausted. Indeed, too many interruptions. And then the phone rang. Another interruption. It was a friend with good news. I felt much better. The next day was a joy. No interruptions. Wrong!

We are creatures who are capable of knowingly interrupting the order of things so that we might better understand the order of things. With the present book, I do just that: interrupt readers' typical way of understanding the nature, scope, and function of interruption. I maintain that interruption is an essential feature of human existence; without the presence of interruption in our lives, we would not be the creatures that we are. In fact, we would not be at all. My assessment of the interruption that we are includes a discussion of its proposed origins, how it forms the existential basis of the health of our lived bodies, how our health is affected when interruptions expose us to the interruption that we are, how the rhetorical construction of narratives provides a way of dealing with the consequences of this exposure, and how these narratives inform instances of public moral argument. The extent of the exposure is dependent on how significant the interruptions are to the health of the lived body. Disaster is always a possibility; the interruption that we are exhibits a destructive and defeatist impulse. Our interruptive nature, however, also exhibits a productive and perfective impulse. The health of the lived body benefits from this function. The rhetorical construction of narratives lends advantage to the function. The benefits extend to others when we use our narratives to help them sustain and improve the health of their lived bodies. I offer a series of case studies in public moral argument that provide concrete illustrations of this ethical, rhetorical, and therapeutic activity.

My assessment of interruption continues my interest in developing a philosophy of communication ethics dedicated to promoting and maintaining our personal and communal well-being. The central phenomena that have so far structured this philosophy include conscience, acknowledgment, the rhetorical creation of discursive openings in interpersonal relationships, and perfection.[1] Interruption plays a role in my investigations of all of these phenomena. The reader who is familiar with my work will see similarities between what I say about interruption in these investigations and what I say about its status in the present project. The similarities serve the goals of ensuring coherency in my ongoing assessment of the topic and facilitating an awareness of differences that mark my past and present treatment of interruption. The similarities are foundational. The differences are both foundational and extensive.

By the time the reader finishes reviewing the introduction, he or she will see clearly that the status I grant interruption qualifies as positing a worldview: a narrative that suggests a way of seeing and interpreting reality. A narrative is a story. I am composing a narrative that tells a story about interruption. The essential elements of these communicative and rhetorical devices are present. A Theme: interruption as an essential feature of existence that incites distress and demise, joy and progress, and discourse. Characters: especially with the case studies there are many, including myself. Settings: as many as there are characters. Conflict: found in the narratives and stories offered by the characters. Plot: the presence of interruption in our lives, how it affects the health of the lived body and encourages the enactment of rhetorical competence, and what will become of the lived body as we increase the life-changing power of interruption.[2]

One final prefatory note. The whole time I was composing my story, I had the following therapeutic words of the philosopher Georges Gusdorf next to my computer. The words speak to the importance of communication, rhetoric, and the health of the lived body: "The decision to express marks the threshold between the passivity of eating one's heart out and creative activity. To speak, to write, to express is to act, to survive crisis, to begin living again, even when one thinks it is only to relive one's sorrow. Expression is a kind of exorcism because it crystallizes the resolve not to let oneself go."[3] The insight offered me nerve and encouragement. I have not always been successful when interruptions brought me face to face with the interruption that we are. The wrong rhetoric was at work. I know more than a few people who can identify with the situation. All of the case studies included in my story raise ethical issues associated with the health of the lived body. I have no doubt that, depending on their stance regarding these issues, readers will find wrong rhetoric at work in some of these cases. Disagreements, of course, still can have educational value. Dealing successfully with the interruption that we are requires stamina and know-how. The interruption never lets up. The health of the lived body is never guaranteed. Rhetorical competence is a needed skill when constructing narratives meant to benefit our well-being. Such competence, at its best, demonstrates the perfective-oriented talent of finding the right words to disclose the truth of the matters at hand. The interruption that we are encourages the cultivation of this talent.

Acknowledgments

I interrupted many people's lives, programs, and institutions as I wrote this book and sought their critical assessments. Many thanks to Pat Arneson; Ron Arnett; Tony Atala; Jarrod Atchison; Michelle Ballif; Wayne Beach; Nathan Bledsoe; Art Bochner; John Bost; Stuart Chambers; Paolo de Coppi; Diane Davis; Jim Denton; Sandy Dickson; Carolyn Ellis; Linda Haines Fogle; Pat Gehrke; Great Ormand Street Hospital (London, England); James Herrick; Ana Iltis; Chris Johnstone; William Kane; Lisa Keränen; Nancy King; Caroline Lee; Andrew Leslie; Lisbeth Lipari; Andrew Lopez; Ananda Mitra; John Moskop; Amit Pinchevski; Ashleigh Rainko; Rich Robeson; Aarti Sarwal; Calvin Schrag; Craig R. Smith; Surgery Unit of Institute of Child Health (London, England); Joe Verga; Eric Watts; Alan Wolfson; Meg Zulick; faculty and staff of The Center for Bioethics, Health, and Society, Wake Forest University School of Medicine; The Institute for Regenerative Medicine, Wake Forest University School of Medicine; The Documentary Film Program, Wake Forest University; Provost Fund, Wake Forest University; Northwestern University School of Medicine; and undergraduate and graduate students in my courses on communication ethics, rhetorical criticism, and health communication and bioethics. I am also grateful to those groups who heard and responded to earlier versions of some of my chapters at the University of Pittsburgh, Duquesne University, Hope College, and conferences sponsored by the National Communication Association. The editorial staff at the University of South Carolina Press proved invaluable, as did two external reviewers whose critiques and generous comments helped me clean up the mess of the draft that they first read. Very special thanks to Mr. Dan Diaz for permission to use the photographs of his wife, Brittany Maynard, and for the conversations he shared with me about her life and death. And then there is my wife, Bobette. I am alive and well owing to her presence in my life.

Introduction

Interrupting Interruption

Interruption is typically conceived as a bothersome and irritating event. This downside of interruption is suggested by dictionary definitions that emphasize how it constitutes a "breaking in" on the "uniformity or continuity" of some thought or action. Here a negative connotation ("breaking in" as a sort of misdemeanor) trumps a positive connotation (the praiseworthiness of consistency). Some interruptions warrant little, if any, concern. While opening the front door to your house, you drop your keys. No big thing. The momentary event doesn't even register as an annoyance, but it certainly is an interruption. The continuity of an action has been delayed. Other interruptions can be more bothersome. If when walking straight to work you trip over a stone and fall and the fall results in a serious injury requiring immediate medical attention, the significance of interruption becomes more remarkable. Then there are interruptions whose presence is a saving grace. Having a friend call you out of a room where you are having a conversation with a person who is boring you to death is a welcomed interruption. Continuity does not always serve us well.

Still, interruptions have a reputation for getting in the way of our thoughts and actions. Studies have shown, for example, that in workplace environments and conversational transactions, interruptions can lower a person's self-confidence, induce stress and anxiety, be employed as a power strategy to dominate, control, and manipulate interpersonal behavior, and violate a speaker's right to voice his or her opinions and arguments. But then again, there is a positive side to interruption. When seen by a speaker as an attempt to keep a dialogue going about the speaker's point of view, overlapping interruptions can enhance cooperative and supportive behavior between the involved parties.[1]

Dialogue, in fact, owes its existence to interruption. Even in a friendly flowing dialogue, the continuity of the conversation is made possible by a turn-taking exchange of talk, and the exchange marks the moment of interruption. Without this moment, we have a soliloquy, not a dialogue. Yet, the person who enjoys being too much of an interruption during a dialogue risks being characterized as a nuisance. Socrates, the self-proclaimed "gadfly," fits the bill. Samuel Beckett's classic tragicomedy *Waiting for Godot,* with its mind-bending dialogue, is filled with interruptions that depict the characters of the play as being nuisances. So, for example, we have this exchange between Estragon, Pozoo, and Vladimir:

> Estragon—"I'm going."
>
> Pozoo—"What was it exactly you wanted to know?"
>
> Vladimir—"Why he—"
>
> Pozoo [angrily]—"Don't interrupt me!" [Pause. Calmer.] "If we all speak at once we'll never get anywhere. [Pause.] "What was I saying?" [Pause. Louder.] "What was I saying?"[2]

Waiting for Godot is its own interruption. Who is Godot? The waiting for whoever this being is interrupts the continuity of whatever else the characters would be doing in their everyday lives. The play also interrupts the audience's conditioned expectations of what a play should be. The play writer Becket is a nuisance.

However, as in the cases of Socrates and Beckett, committed as they are to teaching about the worthiness of seeking the truth and humankind's inexhaustible search for meaning, a nuisance can have good intentions in interrupting a given state of affairs. Another example: In her essay "The Point of the Long and Winding Sentence," Pico Iyer tells us that when she "began writing for a living, my feeling was that my job was to give the reader something vivid, quick and concrete that she couldn't get in any other form; a writer was an information-gathering machine, I thought, and especially as a journalist, my job was to go out into the world and gather details, moments, impressions as visual and immediate as TV." She continues by explaining how "No writer can compete, for speed and urgency, with texts or CNN news flashes or RSS feeds, but any writer can try to give us the depth, the nuances—the 'gaps' that don't show up on many screens. Not everyone wants to be reduced to a sound bite or a bumper sticker." Iyer's reaction to this disrespectful way of treating reality and its witnesses is to become a nuisance by composing long sentences that interrupt readers' ill-conditioned ways of processing and appreciating the written word. I was taken with her effort as I read the following sentences from her essay:

> Enter (I hope) the long sentence: the collection of clauses that is so many-chambered and lavish and abundant in tones and suggestions, that has so much room for near-contradiction and ambiguity and those places in memory or imagination that can't be simplified, or put into easy words, that it allows the reader to keep many things in her head and heart at the same time, and to descend, as by a spiral staircase, deeper into herself and those things that won't be squeezed into an either/or. With each clause,

> we're taken further and further from trite conclusions—or that at least is the hope—and away from reductionism, as if the writer were a dentist, saying "Open wider" so that he can probe the tender, neglected spaces in the reader (though in this case it's not the mouth that he's attending to but the mind).[3]

These sentences make me think of such other advocates of Iyer's prose style as Charles Dickens, James Joyce, and Virginia Woolf, who I suspect might find her interruptive endeavor laudable. On the other hand, those who lost their breath and attention span reading the sentences are likely to be annoyed by Iyer's redeeming compositional practice. Then, again, there are others who would see the wisdom of her intention. For example, the scientist and theologian Pierre Teilhard de Chardin has the beneficial potential of interruption in mind when he notes: "To jolt the individual out of his natural laziness and the rut of habit, and also from time to time to break up the collective frameworks in which he is imprisoned, it is indispensable that he should be shaken and prodded from outside."[4] The philosopher Michel Foucault also speaks favorably of the phenomenon in aligning it with the "role of the intellectual": "to question over and over again what is postulated as self-evident, to disturb people's mental habits, the way they do and think things, to dissipate what is familiar and accepted, to reexamine rules and institutions and on the basis of this re-problematization . . . to participate in the formation of a political will."[5] The physicist, historian, and philosopher of science Thomas Kuhn attests to the power of interruption when he tells us that "scientific revolutions" presuppose a "sense of malfunction" in a given scientific paradigm.[6] The rhetorical theorist and critic Thomas Farrell aligns this power with the orator's art: "Rhetoric, despite its traditional and quite justifiable association with the preservation of cultural truisms, may also perform an act of critical interruption where the taken-for-granted practices of culture are concerned." With the goal of improvement and progress in mind, "[t]he phenomenon of rhetorical interruption juxtaposes the assumptions, norms, and practices of a people so as to prompt a reappraisal of where they are culturally, what they are doing, and where they are going."[7]

These four authors associate interruption with social, political, scientific, and cultural progress. The novelist, poet, literary critic, essayist, lay theologian, and Christian Apologist C. S. Lewis speaks of neither the benefits nor the burdens of interruption but would have us elevate the phenomenon to holy heights: "The great thing, if one can, is to stop regarding all the unpleasant things as interruptions of one's 'own', or 'real' life. The truth is of course that what one calls the interruptions are precisely one's real life—the life God is sending one day by day."[8] I neither affirm nor deny the validity of this last metaphysical claim, although my eventual assessment of the inextricable relation between interruptions and one's real life does encourage such speculation.

Be they appreciated or not, interruptions are here to stay. Our lives begin with an interruption (a sperm fertilizing an egg and a slap on the butt) and end with one, too. In between this beginning and ending, interruptions abound, so much so, in fact, that as a way of coping with their irritating presence we organize them into well-conditioned and taken-for-granted behavioral norms whereby the interruptions lose their disruptive and questioning function as they become ever more a part of our daily routines. But interruption has the last say. The prevalence of text messaging in what the literary theorist David Hillman and the psychoanalyst Adam Phillips term today's "culture of interruption" is a case in point. People have made this one-time interruptive and communicative practice so much a part of their everyday existence that not receiving and sending a text message for too long a time is itself an interruption of the normality of interruptions that are no longer exhibiting a disruptive function. Hillman and Phillips have it right: "Clearly, the whole notion of interruption shows us something about the nature of our commitment to continuity, to sequence, to pattern, to order."[9] This commitment is undeniable. Interruptions make sure of that.

The more one realizes how necessary interruption is to our everyday existence, the more the following counterintuitive contention should make sense: Nothing happens without the force of interruption operating in our lives; the phenomenon must be at work if anything in the world is to be distinguishable and meaningful. For example, angered somewhat by his ten-year-old son's behavior and dismissive attitude toward his parents, a father, seeking more community with his son, desperately pleads with the boy: "Listen to me! I need your undivided attention!" Before the command, the father's identity is made possible by the many other things that interrupt his presence and make his identity distinguishable and meaningful. After the command, if it is heeded, the interruptive force of the father's identity is greatly enhanced, so much so that the interruptive force of other things, although still operative, becomes negligible, disappearing under the influence of an angered father whose interruptive force is now all that matters. If these interruptions were not present, there would be nothing requiring the son's undivided attention, nothing for him to listen to "without interruption." It is not mere difference but rather the force of interruption that makes a difference in the circumstances of everyday life. Identity without difference does not make sense; nor does difference without identity and the force of interruption that brings them together and spreads them apart. The philosopher Jean-Luc Nancy offers a relevant insight related to this point: "Interruption occurs at the edge, or rather it constitutes the edge where beings touch each other, expose themselves to each other and separate from one another, thus communicating and propagating their community."[10]

Here is another way to think about the necessity of interruption: In order for you to read the sentences that I am writing here, you must be able to distinguish words, letters, and punctuation marks from one another. The spaces between all of these figures mark the places that separate and thus interrupt the figures' presence so that they have an identity that is recognized by how it differs from the identity of other letters, words, sentences, and punctuation marks. Without all of these interruptions, there would be nothing to read. Solid black lines and white spaces that separate them would be all that there is to the pages inside a book now void of meaningful content. The philosopher Jacques Derrida agrees: The "caesura ["break" or "interruption" of signs in a text] makes meaning emerge . . . without interruption—between letters, words, sentences, books—no significance could be awakened."[11]

My employment of Derrida warrants further comment. Derrida's claim is based on his notion of "the play of *differance*" that lies at the heart of his philosophy of deconstruction. The play of *differance,* as the linguist Ferdinand de Saussure first emphasized, defines "the basic economy of language": the way in which language functions not only as a semiotic system of differences, of arbitrary and conventionalized signifier/signified relationships and oppositions, but also as a "temporizing" (or "deferring") movement of significations whereby any given semiotic system of meaning, as it takes form, always enters into an "intertextual" relationship with some other (different) system of meaning.[12] Derrida thus claims that "There are only everywhere differences and traces of traces. . . . Nothing—no present and in-*different* being—thus precedes *differance* and spacing."[13] When Derrida, as noted, refers to the necessary interruption between letters, words, sentences, and books, he is speaking about their being separated and thus different from one another. So what is the difference between interruption and *differance*? Is it fair to say that nothing precedes interruption?

Derrida grants *differance* a primordial status. I am suggesting that interruption has a role to play in making sense of *differance.* For the purposes of this project, however, the fundamental relationship of *differance* and interruption is not a guiding concern. Rather, my story about interruption favors an existential appreciation of its nature, scope, and function. The following short story offers some initial guidance to what my longer story entails. The story is based on an actual event that took place during the early stages of writing this book. This story has an unbelievable element to it. But the story is factual.

The call came at 6:30 Sunday morning. I was working at my computer and get quite annoyed by interruptions when I am really into my writing. But the phone displayed a number that I couldn't refuse. It was my dear friend Bo. We go back a long way. He is always there for me. I am always there for him. We're close, tight, brothers in arms.

Bo is brilliant: a B.S. and M.A. in Industrial Administration; rigorous training in electrical engineering, industrial engineering, econometrics; a C.P.A.; a financial analyst; Chief Financial Officer at one of the largest private real estate development agencies in the United States; and a statistician second to none. Being rational is for him all about science, statistics, equations, and spreadsheets. That's a perfect way to be.

The first minute of our conversation was devoted to traditional banter: "Hey, how are you doing?" and things like that. But then he said he had to share an experience he had had the previous night that was "freaking" him out. He sounded excited and a bit anxious. I was about to hear a story about my friend having to deal with a fundamental interruption of existence.

Bo's wife, children, and grandchildren were gathered at his house to celebrate the first night of the Jewish holiday Hanukkah. Bo does not practice the religion. He describes himself as a "Jewish agnostic," whatever that means. Religion is too metaphysical, too irrational. My heritage is Jewish, but I do not practice that or any other organized religion. As an academic, however, I do draw insights from the Bible that I find fitting for my teaching and research projects. When I once was trying to make a point during a past conversation and quoted a sentence from the existential and Christian philosopher Søren Kierkegaard, Bo's immediate and unfriendly response was "Don't give me that academic bullshit."

The only reason Bo was celebrating Hanukkah was for his grandchildren, one of whom was eight years old and wanted to play the holiday-related game dreidel. A dreidel is a four-sided spinning toy. Each side bears a letter of the Hebrew alphabet: *Nun, Gimel, He,* and *Shin.* Together these letters form the acronym Nes Gadol Hayah Sham: "A great miracle happened there" (referring to the Land of Israel). Each player spins the dreidel once during each turn. Depending on which letter appears after a spin, the player wins or loses a game piece associated with the playful activity.

The game began. Bo's spins produced various results. His grandchild's spins produced otherwise, all in a row: I Gimel, then 5, 10, 15, 20, 25, 30, 35, 38. Bo stopped the game, not believing what he was seeing. He hurried to his computer and calculated the probability of spinning thirty-eight successive gimels. Here is the answer: 000000000000000000000132348898008484 percent (one chance in 1.324 sextillion). Bo yelled for the rest of the family to gather around the game and watch what was happening. The spins began again, and the mind-boggling event continued as the child took his turns: 39, 40, 45, 50, 53. Bo couldn't take it anymore. The game stopped. Bo calculated. The probability of spinning fifty-three gimels in a row is 000000000000000000000000000000123260 percent (one chance in 1.233 nonillian).

Bo first described what had happened as "impossible." Then, being the rational person that he is, he corrected himself and admitted that it was "*highly* improbable." But he was emphatic as he swore, "I witnessed the spins. I have the numbers. I am telling the truth. But how could this happen?" Bo's world of know-how could not accommodate what he was experiencing. Simply put for now, a world of know-how is a realm of understanding and meaning; it defines a narrative domain of common sense, habits, routines, rules, beliefs, and stories that are well known for prescribing how we should think and act in appropriate and fulfilling ways. The world of know-how grants structure, order, and direction to what I term the health of the lived body's everyday existence. The lived body is a person having been conditioned by past and present experiences and involvements to know how to think about personal and communal existence and the possibilities for acting in the world. The lived body inhabits a world of know-how and embodies its prescribed ways of managing everyday existence. A person's world of know-how is a place, a habitat, where the person can commune with others who, owing to their worldviews, can think and act like (or at least tolerate) the person. A world of know-how also is an interruption, since this habitat is what it is because its presence interrupts the presence of other worlds of know-how. This interruptive habitat eventually goes unnoticed by its inhabitants once its ways and means of operation become the common sense of everyday life and are taken for granted. The health of the lived body is a function of how well one is faring in a world of know-how. This definition of health involves more than the lived body's "state of physical well-being."[14] Rather, the definition favors the holistic conception of health offered by the World Health Organization (WHO): a "state of complete physical, mental and social well-being and not merely the absence of disease or infirmity."[15] Another word for "complete" is "perfect." The health of the lived body is influenced by how perfect it finds its world of know-how to be.

I reminded Bo that the letters on the dreidel form the acronym for "A great miracle happened there [in Israel]" and that the letter Gimel means a "benefactor" or someone who gives to others. He was adamant as he emphasized that he believed not in miracles "but only in the natural laws of the universe." Nevertheless, his world of know-how had been interrupted, and the health of his lived body was not as perfect as he wanted it to be. He called me because he was all dressed up with numbers and had nowhere to go. His unwavering way of seeing and understanding the world was being interrupted by what he termed the "irrationality" of the symbols (numbers) that made possible his rationale way of seeing and comprehending reality. With his trusted world of know-how in disarray, he nevertheless sounded like he was enjoying himself. The conversation continued as we expressed our amazement over the fifty-four consecutive spins and tried to identify what intervening variables might have influenced the "miraculous" event. It was rewarding. Bo is not a great listener, but his mood provided an opening for me to join him in saying more about this event. The words of the philosopher Karl Jaspers are especially fitting here: "What is not realized in communication is not yet, what is not ultimately grounded in it is without adequate foundation. The truth begins with two."[16]

Wanting to maintain and perhaps expand this opening, I decided to quote Jaspers without telling him that I was doing so. It was a strategic rhetorical maneuver, a minuscule attempt to be eloquent. "You know, Bo, 'Because of the uncertainty of temporal existence life is always an experiment.'"[17] "Uncertainty" and "experiment" are god terms for a person like Bo. Scientists and statisticians make their living by designing experiments to deal with uncertainty and eliminate it as much as possible. "We interest a man by dealing with his interests," writes Kenneth Burke.[18] The maneuver worked. A perfect choice of words. We started to compare the probability of the consecutive spins with cosmological measurements of the universe and, on a more philosophical note, how uncertainty plays such a significant role in our everyday existence. With my book project in mind, I noted that, owing to uncertainty, to the temporal opening we call the future, our self-assured beliefs regarding what we claim to know about ourselves, others, and the world in general are always being called into question. What can happen tomorrow? Who can say for sure? Bo agreed. I then pointed out that a question is an interruption. Again he agreed. It follows then, I said, that human existence is fundamentally an interruption; it never stops putting you and your beliefs to the test, it never ceases bringing to mind the issue of contingency. The interruption that we are is a question always being asked: Are you sure? Are you sure? Are you sure? The questioning function of our existence is a reality check: It challenges us to perfect our capacity to know and express the truth of matters of concern. The interruption that we are calls us to be open-minded, virtuous, dignified, and skilled in having a truthful way with words. It is as if we have been given a gift to be good. The gift is a given, an a priori condition of existence. Bo remained silent, which worried me a bit. But I continued, noting that Kierkegaard had coined an oxymoron to describe our interruptive nature when formulating his religious beliefs: "objective uncertainty." Bo chuckled, but he didn't call it academic bullshit. Rather, he was taken with the use of an interruptive figure of speech to disclose the interruption that we are. I then said something like this: "When the spins interrupted your world of know-how, Bo, you were exposed to this interruption. The exposure has good and bad consequences, depending on how well you deal with it. The interruption that we are exhibits a perfective function. It calls for concerned thought and action that enables you to deal with and perhaps improve and perfect as much as possible the health of your lived body. Our conversation is a case in point."

We continued to say a few more words about uncertainty and, now with Kierkegaard in mind, religion, too, and we eventually got to a point where the spins came up again and Bo admitted that while witnessing the event he felt like "Moses looking at the burning bush." Now this admission was not as improbable as one chance in 1.233 nonillian, but it still was stunning. We recalled the actor Charlton Heston's role in the famous movie *The Ten Commandments,* and

I asked Bo if his face turned a shade of grey as he listened to what the burning spins had to say. It was a good laugh for both of us.

The narrative had changed: statistics, science, philosophy, cosmology, and now religion. Bo asked me whether I thought something spiritual had been going on with his grandchild and his witnessing of the spins. That wasn't for me to say. The decision was his to make. Our conversation was not meant to persuade; rather, it was intended to enhance a communal bond between friends who put their egos aside in favor of trying to disclose as much as possible the truth of the matter at hand. We were engaged in the rhetorical construction of a narrative that had a variety of components and whose final structure had yet to be determined.

Bo and I had been talking for nearly two hours. It was time to say adieu. Before hanging up the phone, however, I asked him to do me one favor: You need not abandon your long-standing world of know-how, but please try to stay open to what you witnessed. Take time to ponder it some more. Open-mindedness is the key. The uncertainty of existence calls you to do so. Be true to that call. Science does it. The ethic of science requires its practitioners to stay open to the data in the name of truth. The same ethic lies at the heart of religion. In order to witness God's presence (whatever or whomever that is), one must stay open to how that presence is showing itself in the happenings of life. Both science and religion value perfection. The next time we talk, educate me. I will not bring up the topic again unless you initiate the discussion.

Bo remains a brilliant statistician housed in the world of high finance. I am convinced that, like me, he will never forget our conversation and the event that initiated it. Interrupting narratives had emerged to deal with the interruption that we are. How much of them he took to heart remains a question. The health of his lived body will be a determining factor. Having to confront the interruption that we are can be as disconcerting as it is rewarding. It's a matter of how well you can handle a question that comes not from the mouth of another human being. We did not create the spatial-temporal structure of existence that opens us to the future and with its uncertainty calls us into question. Sometimes you need help in dealing with this uncertainty. Sometimes you don't.

An interruption that interrupted an interruptive domain of know-how started this whole process. A third and more fundamental interruption—the interruption that we are—then showed itself. A fourth interruption was needed as a possible way of handling the "narrative wreckage" at hand.[19] This fourth interruption involved the rhetorical construction of a narrative that interrupted the third interruption so to reestablish the interruptive domain of a world of know-how where the lived body could regain a sense of feeling secure and at home with itself, others, and its immediate surroundings. My experience with Bo consisted of five interruptions. The relevance of worlds of know-how—statistics, science, philosophy, cosmology, and religion—was on the line, as was the health of his lived body. The philosopher William Earle associates this state of being of the lived body with the "nostalgia for something final and absolute," something as complete and perfect as possible.[20] This description is especially appropriate for my purposes in that the desire being identified—"nostalgia," from the Greek *nostos:* to return home—speaks of that existential condition where one feels "homeless" and is thus "homesick." It is an unhealthy and imperfect way to be. That's why Bo called me. That's why he was open to the narratives of worlds of know-how other than his own. That's why he was willing to become engaged in the rhetorical construction of a narrative that could help him contend with his being exposed to the interruption that we are. It was a matter of reinstating a degree of completeness and perfection to the health of a lived body. Indeed, the interruption that we are is a gift to be good. We are fortunate creatures, and pitiful, too, given how often throughout history this gift has been put to disgraceful use.

For the fun of it, I imagined Bo, after much deliberation, going back to his high-finance world of know-how, sharing our narrative with his colleagues, and employing his way with words to make clear that he was convinced that what he had witnessed with his grandson's spinning of the dreidel was a spiritual event, a sign of something much greater than anything that went on every day in his technical business environment. As he stood his ground against those who thought he was out of his mind, the communicative transaction would qualify as a well-worth-seeing instance of public moral argument.[21]

My assessment of interruption deals with all that I have said about my experience with Bo. If there had been more time to talk and if I had thought Bo were willing to listen, I would have said more about the nature, scope, and function of our interruptive nature. Now, however, is the appropriate time to do so. Some additional introductory remarks about this matter will be helpful in orienting the reader to the narrative structure of my story.

Our well-being and survival are dependent on our ability to respond to the dynamics of our interruptive nature with concerned thought and decisive action. Sometimes lived bodies don't make it. I have stood face to face with the interruption that we are a time or two. Uncertainty is the source of anxiety, and this emotion can be crushing. I learned what it takes to survive. The wounds never completely go away. I know a number of people who would agree. I suspect there are many more. If you can construct some narrative that can start rebuilding a world of know-how, then, indeed, more power to you. Nietzsche is right: "What does not kill me makes me stronger."[22] If you have somebody willing to help you construct the narrative, count your blessings.

In order to be as truthful as possible, the rhetorical construction of narratives must make use of what the cultural critic and rhetorical theorist Kenneth

Burke describes as the "perfectionist impulse" of language. According to Burke, "The principle of perfection is central to the nature of language as motive. The mere desire to name something by its 'proper' name, or to speak a language in its distinctive ways is intrinsically 'perfectionist.' What is more 'perfectionist' in essence than the impulse, when one is in dire need of something, to so state this need that one in effect 'defines' the situation?"[23] We are creatures who would enhance and better (perfect) our understanding of the world in order to live wise and fulfilling lives. To define what something is, is to engage in an act of truth telling, of telling it like *it is.* Truth happens first and foremost as a disclosing of the world, a revealing of something that directs our concern (for example, a flower blooming). Any truth claim (such as "That rose is in bloom") presupposes this act of disclosure. Truth shows itself in narratives that warrant praise for being revelatory and perhaps even awe-inspiring because of the way they call forth and disclose their subject matter, thereby enabling us to perfect our understanding and appreciation of what is being talked about.

The practice of rhetoric involves, among other things, finding a way with words that facilitates this revelatory process. The process brings about the interruptive nature of our worlds of know-how. In order for this disclosing function of language to be successful, it must also operate to indicate what the matters under consideration *are not.* As the philosopher Hans Jonas reminds us: "the capacity for truth presupposes the capacity to negate. . . . [O]nly a being that can entertain negativity . . . can entertain truth."[24] Negating is an act of interruption: distinguishing one thing from another. The identity of anything (for example, a particular world of know-how) necessities an appreciation of difference. The rhetorical construction of a narrative intended to disclose the truth puts a lot of pressure on those who are up for the task.

Indeed, rhetoric's ability to find ways of communicating the truth when constructing narratives defines an ethical endeavor that grants this practical art well-deserved respectability. Within the rhetorical tradition, this endeavor defines the "art of eloquence" (*oratio*): the ability to equip (*ornare*) knowledge of a subject in such a way that it can assume a publicly accessible form and function effectively in the social and political arena. The art of eloquence facilitates the righteous quality of public moral argument. The ancient Roman rhetorical theorist Cicero has this point in mind when he writes: "[W]hat function is so kingly, so worthy of the free, so generous, as to bring help to the suppliant, to raise up those who are cast down, to bestow security, to set free from peril, to maintain men in their civil rights? . . . The wise control of the complete orator is that which chiefly upholds not only his own dignity, but the safety of countless individuals and of the entire State."[25] The interruptive nature of existence never ceases to question how truthful we are in making the world meaningful. Of course, whatever one person claims to be the truth, another person can see that truth claim as deficient, deceitful, and perhaps dangerous. The rhetoric that facilitates the perfectionist impulse of language is oftentimes faced with a challenging endeavor.

All that I am saying about rhetoric is accounted for by the transcendentalist Ralph Waldo Emerson when he writes of the heroic nature of the orator's art: "Certainly there is no true orator who is not a hero. . . . The orator must ever stand with forward foot, in the attitude of advancing. . . . His speech is not to be distinguished from action. It is action, as the general's word of command or shout of battle is action."[26] This claim calls into question a well-known maxim of our culture—"Actions speak louder than words"—that is famous for its "put-down" of the practice of rhetoric. The metaphor that informs the eloquence of Emerson's claim lends it further force for, indeed, heroes and war are readily related. When Emerson speaks of the true orator's heroism, however, his understanding of "war" emphasizes what he terms "a military attitude of the soul" that is not directed toward the actual killing of others. Instead, this attitude is needed by the orator who would "dare the gibbet and the mob," the rage and retribution of a misinformed and closed-minded public, when attempting to move its members beyond the blinders of their "commonsense" beliefs and toward a genuine understanding of what, for the orator, is arguably the truth of some immediate matter of concern. For Emerson, the heroism and dignity of the true orator are made possible not only by his "power to connect his thought with its proper symbol, and so to utter it" but also, and primarily, by his "love of truth and . . . [the] desire to communicate it without loss."[27] The process presupposes the imaginative capacity of the orator to construct dwelling places for his or her audience, to create openings for others that allow for collaborative deliberation about the truth of the matters at hand. I agree with the literary critic Northrop Frye: "As long as a single form of life remains in misery and pain the imagination finds the world not good enough."[28] The heroic nature of the true orator entails moral obligations.

I like to think of the worthiness and stunning difficulty of meeting these moral obligations with the words of one of my favorite authors, Annie Dillard, in mind: "Write as if you were dying. At the same time, assume you write for an audience consisting solely of terminal patients. That is, after all, the case. What would you begin writing if you knew you would die soon? What could you say to a dying person that would not enrage by its triviality?" . . . "Why are we reading, if not in hope of beauty laid bare, life heightened and its deepest mystery probed?"[29] Dillard's questions interrupt my life as a writer. They are meant to do the same to anyone who takes on the challenge of demonstrating the needed rhetorical skill to disclose the truth in a way that will inspire others. Practice makes perfect, so they say. Athletic coaches and trainers are fond of amending this saying: "Perfect practice makes perfect." I have been practicing my entire professional life. It never ends. The interruption is always there. The myth of Sisyphus for real.

Interruptions are a fact of life that happens for good and ill. Jaspers associates the latter alternative with what he terms "the desire to lead a philosophical life." This desire "springs from the darkness in which the individual finds himself, from his sense of forlornness when he stares without love into the void, from his self-forgetfulness when he feels that he is being consumed by the busyness of the world, when he suddenly wakes up in terror and asks himself: What am I, what am I failing to do, what should I do?"[30] Given what I have said so far about interruption, I agree with Jaspers, especially when I keep in mind that the interruptive situation he is referring to has redemptive force. I, however, would add another question to the one cited by Jaspers. Coming face to face with our interruptive nature, a person, during and after his or her journey to the heart of existence, may wonder in a philosophical moment: "Why is existence structured as an interruption?" Indeed, given the way it functions, the interruption that we are calls into question its own way of being. Nevertheless, there it is. Without the interruption that we are, no other interruptions that take place in our everyday existence would exist. No play of *differance* either. The question remains unanswered. So we still have reason to wonder. "Why" questions are in search of a source that caused our predicament. It's a matter of history, of discovering beginnings, which once discovered might nevertheless encourage more wondering. Do beginnings have beginnings? The words of the philosopher Ludwig Wittgenstein come to mind: "It is so difficult to find the beginning. Or, better, it is difficult to begin at the beginning. And not try to go further back."[31]

The topic of interruption, especially as the phenomenon forms the fundamental basis of our existence, encourages us to go further back. We can measure and calculate the spatiotemporal operation of our interruptive nature with such devices as clocks, calendars, and maps. But this transformation of the operation does not account for the actual presence and dynamics of the spatiotemporal function of the interruption that we are—the way this phenomenon happens *before* it is transformed into measurable instants, the way it opens us to the contingency and uncertainty of the future. Human being is *more* than we make of it through our daily activities; there is an "otherness" that lies at the heart of our existence. The interruption that we are is nothing without this otherness. The engineer, architect, and inventor R. Buckminster Fuller speaks of the relationship as "the a priori mystery, within which consciousness first formulates and from which enveloping and permeating mystery consciousness never completely separates, but which it often ignores then forgets altogether or deliberately disdains." Fuller would thus have us realize that "consciousness begins as an awareness of otherness, which otherness awareness requires time.

And all statements by consciousness are in the comparative terms of prior observations of consciousness ('It's warmer, it's quicker, it's bigger than the other or others'). Minimal consciousness evokes time, as a nonsimultaneous sequence of experiences. Consciousness dawns with the second experience. This is why consciousness identified the basic increment of time as being a second. Not until the second experience did time and consciousness combine as human life."[32]

The second experience referred to qualifies as an interruption—a break in the continuity of sameness by otherness. Assessing the interruption that we are demands that the phenomenon of otherness be acknowledged as much as possible, even if it forces us to move from everyday empirical existence to the realm of metaphysics.

The Judeo-Christian tradition of religion and the science of cosmology attune us to this otherness as they teach us, respectively, about God's relationship with humankind and the related theories of the big bang and the eternal inflation of the cosmos. These teachings offer explanations of what was going on in the beginning. And, importantly, they also point to interruption as playing a fundamental role in this remarkable event. The nature, scope, and function of interruption have a long history. In the beginning was an interruption. The interruption that we are came after that. Chapter 1 offers an account of the origins of interruption and how it materializes itself on earth, becoming the interruption that we are. My interpretation of what religion and science have to say about these matters demonstrates that, right from the beginning, the life of interruption shows itself to be a robust phenomenon.

The interruption that we are makes itself known in the world of everyday existence, marked as it is by the ever-present uncertainty of the future. My existential approach to investigating the interruption includes a phenomenological assessment of the topic. The three philosophers who are supportive of this type of analysis and who I find most instructive for developing an understanding of the nature, scope, and function of our interruptive nature include Søren Kierkegaard, Martin Heidegger, and Emmanuel Levinas. The combined works of these philosophers is, to say the least, extensive. With what I have to say about their writings, I intend to be particularly selective in identifying and interrelating relevant material that facilitates the construction of my story. Kierkegaard's and Heidegger's respective analyses of the interruption that we are focus primarily on the perfectiveness of the self's existence. The analyses are complementary and, in my judgment, best understood by combining them in one chapter (chapter 2). I conclude that chapter with a brief case study of Heidegger's infamous 1933 rectorial address at Freiburg University. My critique of the address emphasizes the disastrous effects that follow from Heidegger's deficient appraisal of the ethical and rhetorical relationship between the self and the other. The critique heads us in the direction of Levinas's philosophy, which emphasizes how the self, in being as perfect as it can be, has an ethical obligation to serve the other. The benefits of this philosophy and certain problems that it raises concerning the self-other relationship are extensive enough to warrant their own chapter (chapter 3). I offer a brief case study that involves these problems. The study focuses on a diary that was written by a Jewish victim of the Holocaust. The narrative of the diary speaks of the diarist's rhetorical struggle to "find the right words" for composing a narrative that helps her understand the health of her lived body and its circumstances and eventually becomes a source for advancing public moral argument about her ordeal. The struggle displays a perfective intent. Kierkegaard, Heidegger, and Levinas omit any detailed discussion of what such a struggle entails. Their work favors theory over practice. The interruption that we are, however, is without a doubt a practical matter. The self's and the other's own existence confirm as much.

Remaining true to the trajectory of my story, I use its final four chapters to present additional case studies that offer a more detailed and practically oriented examination of the central topics of this book. Chapters 4 through 6 involve selves who, like the diarist referred to in my discussion of Levinas, have been exposed to the interruption that we are and have engaged in the rhetorical struggle of constructing narratives to cope with their situations and to perfect as much as possible the health of their lived bodies. The interruption that instigated this state of affairs is illness. This specific interruption is notorious for bringing the lived body face to face with the interruption that we are. The physician and narrative ethics scholar Rita Charon addresses the power of illness and the sickness it produces: "Sickness opens doors. It may not always have been the case, but today, it is more likely to be sickness than, say, the loss of faith that propels a person toward self-knowledge and clarifying of life goals and values. It is when you are sick that you have to question whom in your life you trust, how much life means to you, how much suffering you can bear." Moreover, Charon emphasizes that narrative ethics emphasizes "the fundamentally moral [and rhetorical] undertaking of selecting words" that display the evocative power to disclose the reality of the ill person's lived body as it contends with its interruptive nature.[33] The interruption that we are, illness and its physical, social, and personal effects (the health of the lived body), and the rhetorical concerns of narrative ethics go together.

Along with a growing number of researchers in medicine, bioethics, and health communication, Charon's influential teaching and research program in narrative ethics focuses on the communicative dynamics of the physician-patient-family member encounter. Research in narrative ethics is not, however, restricted to this interpersonal setting. The well-being of the body politic of democracy requires that issues related to the health of the lived body transcend the institutional boundaries of the medical establishment in order to educate the citizenry about these issues. This instructional endeavor encourages the production of whatever public moral argument may be necessary to accomplish this task. The cases presented in chapters 4 through 6 are instances of public moral argument that take form as people tell stories about their illnesses for the purpose of advocating ways of respecting and advancing the health of their and others' lived bodies. This particular approach to the study of narrative ethics and health communication extends their range of inquiry, thereby answering calls from health-care professionals and, most recently, the President's Commission for the Study of Bioethical Issues (May 2016) to promote and develop the civic-minded practice of public moral argument.[34]

As seen in the first three cases, the demonstration of this practice is displayed in stories about how the symbolism of a single word enhances an appreciation of the role that compassion plays in the life of a patient suffering from heart disease (chapter 4); how a disability rights activist must defend her personhood against a distinguished and controversial university professor who advocates the practices of eugenics and euthanasia (chapter 5); and how a young woman dying from brain cancer must defend her decision, against staunch opposition, to opt for the procedure of medical aid in dying (chapter 6). Storytelling as a form of public moral argument is what the rhetorical theorist and critic Walter Fisher has in mind when he tells us that this form of argument "is publicized, made available for consumption and persuasion of the polity at large," and "is aimed at what Aristotle called 'untrained thinkers,' or, to be effective, it should be. Most important, *public* moral argument is a form of controversy that inherently crosses professional fields. It is not contained, in the way that legal, scientific, or theological arguments are, by subject matter, particular conceptions of argumentative competence, and well-recognized rules of advocacy."[35] The first three stories that inform and advance my story function in these ways.

The progression of the stories encourages consideration of what constitutes the "good life." Recall that the interruption that we are can be read empirically as a gift of goodness. Goodness is perfection in the making. The stories speak to the relevance and difficulty of this endeavor and how it necessarily involves a consideration of virtue. Specific virtues that are relevant to my story are initially identified when discussing the philosophies of Kierkegaard, Heidegger, and Levinas. Working together, the stories set the stage for the final case study, which focuses on the public moral arguments that inform the current debate over the benefits and burdens of what is termed our "posthuman future" (chapter 7).

Posthumanity places us face to face with the interruption that we are and offers a narrative of progress that promotes the worldview that goodness is perfection in the making. Posthumanity heralds biotechnological achievements that allow us to reengineer, enhance, and perfect the physical and mental capabilities of our lived bodies beyond what is considered "normal." With the evolution of posthumanity, we increase our ability to heed a particularly significant biblical command—one that, with great economy, says it all when it comes to our purpose on earth and the need to cultivate virtuous behavior: "Walk before me and be thou perfect" (Genesis 17:1).[36] Posthumanity is a source of awe, in both senses of the term: fear and wonder. Critics of posthumanity see it fostering the illness of being rotten with perfection.[37] Advocates of posthumanity see their critics fostering the illness of being rotten with imperfection. Various degrees of these illnesses are identified in the first three cases.

The debate over our posthuman future is concerned with the overall health of our lived body. In this debate there is storytelling going on for untrained thinkers. The storyteller who receives special attention in my discussion of posthumanity is Dr. Francis Collins, who led the team that discovered the language of the human genome and declared it to be "the language of God." Collins also contributes to the more professionally-oriented public moral argument that structures the debate. The rhetorical construction of competing narratives that inform the debate over our posthuman future continues at a rapid pace. The bottom line for these narratives can be stated as a question: Should there be a limit to how far we go in making use of the perfective impulse of the interruption that we are to enhance our physical and mental capabilities? Ray Kurzweil, one of the world's leading inventors and futurists and known in the worlds of computer science, genetics, nanotechnology, robotics, and artificial intelligence as "the restless genius," takes offense at limits when it comes to human enhancement. The perfective impulse of the interruption that we are is supposedly destined for greatness beyond belief. Or, as Kurzweil puts it: "Is there a God? Not yet."[38] The interruption that we are is fated to be interrupted by an interruption: a posthuman being that will rid itself of what once was its interruptive nature. Really?

The story I tell about the interruption that we are remains unfinished. The interruption demands as much. There is no way to determine how long it will take for our postmodern future to materialize fully, or even whether it should. One of my cherished mentors, the philosopher Calvin Schrag, comments on the necessity of such an outcome: "[I]n designing our projects, we need to be mindful that they remain works in progress. They are always provisional and open-ended, with the attached caveat, 'until further notice.' Ourselves and our projects are never finished. When we die, we die unfinished, and so do our projects."[39] Yet, in remaining unfinished, my story still abides by a belief that Schrag instills in his students and that the award-winning poet Brian Christian states so eloquently: "What we are fighting for, in the twenty-first century, is the continued existence of conclusions not already forgone—the continued relevance of judgment and discovery and figuring out, and the ability to continue to exercise them."[40] I read these words as a call for the cultivation of wisdom, which certainly is a goal of this book. Again, the interruption that we are demands as much. Thus my story about this essential feature of human existence.

CHAPTER 1

The First Interruption

> "Science tries to document the factual character of the natural world, and to develop theories that coordinate and explain these facts. Religion, on the other hand, operates in the equally important, but utterly different, realm of human purposes, meanings, and values—subjects that the factual domain of science might illuminate, but can never resolve."
>
> Stephen Jay Gould, *Rocks of Ages*

Where did we come from? When did it all begin? And why? And how? Human beings are obsessed with beginnings. This obsession is driven by a desire to know as much as possible about who we are as inhabitants of the universe. We seek completeness in our lives. Another word for completeness is perfection. More often than not, "good enough" will do for most people. But good enough is not good enough for those whose calling requires them to get to the heart of the matter, to the beginning of it all. It's a long journey. Anthropologists, archeologists, and historians, for example, are invaluable in getting us under way. Religion scholars, philosophers, and cosmologists keep us going. Their professional training obliges them to do so. Their ending is the beginning. Philosophers inform their colleagues that the journey is likely to be an endless task. The philosopher Martin Heidegger's consideration of the matter is a case in point. Although what he has to say regarding the beginning may require more than one reading to deal with his way with words, his insight is instructive:

> The beginning does not at first allow itself to emerge as beginning but instead retains in its own inwardness its beginning character. The beginning then first shows itself in the begun, but even there never immediately and as such. Even if the begun appears as the begun, its beginning and ultimately the entire "essence" of the beginning can still remain veiled. Therefore the beginning first unveils itself in what has already come forth from it. As it begins, the beginning leaves behind the proximity of its beginning essence and in that way conceals itself. Therefore an experience of what is at the beginning by no means guarantees the possibility of thinking the beginning itself in its essence. The first beginning is, to be sure, what

> is decisive for everything; still, it is not the primordial beginning, i.e., the beginning that simultaneously illuminates itself and its essential domain and in that way begins.[1]

Religion and science remain undeterred.

Please keep in mind that the following discussion of religion is not intended as an argument for the correctness of its worldview. I am telling a story about the interruption that we are, and religion demands attention given what it says about the topic. When I turn my attention to science, the story changes dramatically.

Religion

The Bible begins with a story about the beginning, with the first interruption to ever happen: "In the beginning God created the heaven and the earth. And the earth was without form, and void; and darkness was upon the face of the deep. And the Spirit of God moved upon the face of the waters. And God said, Let there be light and there was light" (Genesis 1:1–3). Put another way, God interrupted a state of nothingness and thereby brought about a state of somethingness. The power of interruption became an instructive force of the universe. God makes use of this force, for example, with a simple question directed at Adam, who, having broken God's law against apple-eating, was attempting to hide from sight: "Where art thou?" (Genesis 3:9). Questions are interruptive in nature. They break the continuity of some action or event (for example, hiding) and encourage pause for thought. In Adam's case, the pause was quick: "Here I am!"

The philosopher Hans-Georg Gadamer has this to say about the interruptive function of questions: "The essence of the *question* is to open up possibilities and keep them open. . . . To ask a question means to bring into the open. The openness of what is in question consists in the fact that the answer is not settled. . . . Every true question requires this openness."[2] God's question certainly brought Adam into the open, but his possibilities were already determined. There was no room for further conversation. God's question is rhetorical; it's a call for confession. This is not to say, however, that God's question totally fails the test of being a "true question." The question leaves open the possibility of *choosing* to answer a call, which Adam does when he confesses, "Here I am!" With this confession Adam acknowledges the presence and power of God. God calls for acknowledgment throughout the Bible. The act of acknowledgment is what enables us to open ourselves to whomever or whatever God is and to remain open to the One who on the sixth day of creation acknowledged the worth of bringing humankind into being. What God gave us is what God wants in return. God's rhetorical question to Adam is an interruption that serves a legitimate purpose.

The Judeo-Christian tradition makes much of how "interruption is God's invitation" to awaken us from the everyday routines that blind us to the ways of self-improvement and serving others.[3] If only for a moment, interruptions grant us time to heed God's command "Walk before me and be thou perfect." Christ repeats the command in his sermon on the mount: "Be ye therefore perfect, even as your Father which is in heaven is perfect" (Matthew 5:48). The command is meant to interrupt the lives of those who walk the "crooked paths" of sin (Isaiah 59:8). And notice, too, that the command itself contains an interruption. In order to abide by the command, we need to answer an essential question raised by the command: What exactly is perfection? The command doesn't say. It's an open question. It's debatable. In Gadamer's terms, it's a "true question." The One who makes the command calls for acknowledgment. Are we acknowledging God as we struggle to answer the question and as we most likely interrupt each other in the process, believing at least for the moment that we can offer the best possible response? Why else would God make a command that leaves a crucial term undefined? The meaning of perfection is ambiguous. Ambiguity is a rhetorical device that encourages discussion and debate and the practice of rhetoric, which facilitates these communicative transactions. The need for public moral argument is born. God's command regarding perfection places us in a rhetorical situation. Indeed, as the philosopher Hans Blumenberg points out, "Lacking definitive evidence and being compelled to act are the prerequisites of the rhetorical situation."[4] We have been interrupted by rhetoric that calls for additional rhetoric intended to decipher the truth and tell the story of perfection. The need for the rhetorical construction of a narrative is born.

Rhetoric is at work whenever language is employed to *open* people to ideas, positions, and circumstances that, if rightly understood, stand a better than even chance of getting people to think and act wisely. Orators are forever attempting to create these openings, for this is how they maximize the chance that the members of some audience will take an interest in what is being said and thus become more involved in judging the truthfulness of the orator's discourse. Neither persuasion nor collaborative deliberation can take place without the formation of this joint interest. Interests take form only to the extent that we develop emotional attachments to things happening in our environments. Aristotle offers the first detailed analysis of this fact of life in Book Two of his *Rhetoric*. The rhetorical practice of moving ideas to people and people to ideas is dependent on the ability of orators to attune their discourse to the emotional character of those being addressed.

Acknowledgment happens as the orator is successful in accomplishing this interest-developing activity. The good speaker is always seeking acknowledgment from some audience whose good members are also waiting for the speaker to acknowledge their interests in some meaningful way. In short, rhetorical competence has a significant role to play in providing places (openings) where acknowledgment can be received and, in the best of possible worlds, the truth can be told. To tell the truth is to make the best possible use of the perfectionist impulse of language. Rabbi David Wolpe has this point in mind in telling the story of Moses: "Moses has to wrench words from inside himself. He cannot simply summon the phrase that would placate and please. Rather than the gentle comfort of rolling phrases and smooth oratory, God's leader has to prove by his inner struggle that he shares the people's plight. The leader must also have a catch in his throat, not spread ready rhetoric like a salve over all wounds. Moses cannot lead by means of the easy fluency of the demagogue. His is a hard-earned eloquence. His is less the mastery of the word than the heroism of the word."[5]

Hard-earned eloquence: I understand this to mean a form of rhetorical competence that one acquires not simply by knowing and talking theory but instead by being open and devoted to God's call and willing to enact the effort that it takes to spread the word in a convincing and honest way. Moses is set on a path where the acquisition of rhetorical competence must take place in the practical world of everyday existence.

Rhetorical competence is called for by the interruptive nature of God's command regarding perfection. Left undefined, perfection, and all that it entails, becomes a matter open for debate. As the debate begins and progresses, the One who created this opening with an all-important question receives acknowledgment. To participate in the debate is to say "Here I am" to God. Participants also receive acknowledgment as they feel good about what they are doing. God makes possible this feeling, having gifted human beings with the capacity to appreciate the goodness of their actions. God tells us what this gift is: "I will give them a heart to know me, that I am the Lord" (Jeremiah 24:7). The gift is otherwise known as "conscience" (Latin: *conscientia: con* [with] *scientia* [knowing]), a gift that facilitates a knowing-with God about matters of importance (for example, perfection). Moreover, gifted with a heart, our lived bodies provide God a "dwelling place" (Hebrew: *makom*) where God's presence can be felt in times of need.[6] The health of the lived body is born, as is living a good life.

The more wholehearted people are when engaging in activities that enable them to experience the presence of God in their lives, the more they can feel good about their efforts. Judaism emphasizes the importance of being wholehearted. The Hebrew word for this particular emotional capacity of the lived body is *tamin,* whose primary meaning is "perfection." Dealing with the question of perfection in a wholehearted manner is a perfect thing to do. The effort is a demonstration of what is being called for when God commands, "Walk before me and be thou perfect." The interruptive nature of this command is educational. God is teaching us how emotion and acknowledgment are related and how this relationship can have a positive effect on the health of the lived body.

Rhetoric plays an important role in achieving this result. God employs the rhetorical device of ambiguity to initiate the interruption that makes us wonder about all that perfection entails.

I think it is fair to say that what is going on here is a particular use of the perfectionist impulse of language, the use of the right word, to perfect our ability to understand what God is said to be: perfection. And all of this being the case, I also think it is fair to say that God warrants acknowledgment for demonstrating a high level of rhetorical competence. God is an orator of the first degree. Following God's ways, we thus have an obligation to perfect our ability to be rhetorically competent; interruptions that necessitate the performance of this skill can happen anytime. Fulfilling the obligation also requires knowing how to make the best possible use of the perfectionist impulse of language. With God as our audience, not considering this matter is out of the question. The truth of perfection, of God, is on the line.

Those whose faith is based on a literal interpretation of Scripture are likely to find what I am saying about interruption, God, and perfection to be inappropriate and unneeded. They might say something like this: "To be perfect in God's eyes, just do what God says and does. It's all there in the Bible." So members of a Pentecostal church in the mountains of North Carolina, my home state, live by the word of God recorded in Mark 16:18: "They shall take up serpents." And in Luke 10:19, these snake handlers are reassured that "nothing shall by any means hurt you." Last year a leader of the church was bitten by a snake while holding it during a service. Luke 10:19 didn't work. So much for a perfect reading of the Bible. And while the man lay dying in agony, he refused any treatment because that was not God's way. Where does God say that? With all due respect to his family and fellow church members, the question of perfection is still up for grabs. And then consider this. The story of Noah and the ark tells of how God acted early on when God took exception to the sinful ways of humankind. And God declared, "I will destroy man whom I have created from the face of the earth . . . for it repenteth me that I have made [him]" (Genesis 6:57). The flood came, and humankind was extinguished. There is a word for what God practiced: eugenics. It makes me cringe to say it, given the term's horrendous history, but that's what God chose to do. Speak about an interruption. God was the first eugenicist. Must we do what God did in order to be perfect? The ancient Greek term for eugenics is *eu* (good) *genes* (birth). With this understanding of the term, one could say that God extinguished humankind so to bring about a better breed of humankind. Still, God is a eugenicist. Just how sinful were our ancestors to warrant mass murder? Personally, I would like to hear a bit more debate about what a perfect interruption is.

I am telling a story about interruption. The Judean-Christian tradition tells us the story begins with God's interrupting creation of all there is. There would be no reason to turn to the Judean-Christian religion when telling my story if, in the beginning, God was content with God's own perfection and left well enough alone. The nineteenth-century philosopher Frederick W. J. Schelling has this possibility in mind when he asks: "Has creation a final purpose at all, and if so why is it not attained immediately, why does perfection not exist from the very beginning?"[7] For Schelling, the answer is clear. Perfection takes time: "God is a *life*, not a mere being. All life has a destiny and is subject to suffering and development. God freely submitted himself to this too, in the very Beginning. . . . All history remains incomprehensible without the concept of a humanly suffering God. Scripture, too, . . . puts that time into a distant future when God will be all in all, that is, when He will be completely realized. For this is the final purpose of creation: that which could not be in itself, shall be in itself."[8]

Schelling holds to an evolutionary metaphysics: the notion of an evolving God who has it all together but still needs the thinking and acting of human creatures in order to complete the task of all being One with the cosmos. An earlier version of this theory is developed in the Judaic tradition of Kabbalah (the mystical core of Judaism and ultimately of Christianity and Islam). The theory is based on the teachings of the sixteenth-century rabbi Isaac Luria. His interpretations of the five books of Moses and the *Zohar* (a mystical commentary on these books) give rise to a cosmological myth intended to clarify the workings of the self-manifestation of divinity and how human beings come to play a fundamental role in sustaining this holy happening. The myth calls into question the fundamental belief of older rabbinic theology that God's own well-being is not contingent on human action. Luria insists, on the contrary, that the Creator does need our help. Luria thus creates a new narrative that redefines the traditional understanding of God's perfection. In so doing, he provides an appreciation of interruption that differs significantly from a traditional Christian understanding of the matter. A brief summary of Luria's teachings is sufficient for my purposes.[9]

According to Luria, the Creator's first act was not the interruptive event of "revelation" but rather withdrawal, the creation of an opening, a "void" or empty place within the Creator's infinite presence and perfection. *Ein Sof*, the "endless light" of the Creator, withdrew "from Itself into Itself" in order to make room in the midst of Itself for the entire cosmos to come into being. This act of withdrawal is the Creator interrupting Itself. The action is the ultimate act of self-effacement. Otherness is granted priority in God's workings, a giving way to a place, an infinite dimension of space-time, which allows for life and its development. The essential nature of the Creator is that of sharing and compassion, a desire to give of Itself. This entire process occurs before God's interrupting avowal "Let there be light!" The creation of the cosmos presupposes a more primordial creation: with the Creator's withdrawal there arises an absence, a "nothingness," a vacated place where something other than God can flourish under God's care. Only then can God's next interruption occur.

Luria teaches that before this second interruption took place a crisis occurred in God's creation process. The result of this crisis becomes evident when Moses first stands in God's light and is told that the Jewish people have a future. When Moses asks for God's "Name," he is told, "*Ehyeh-asher-ehyeh.*" English renders this reply in a static way: "I *am* who I *am.*" In Hebrew, however, the dynamic of being open to the future is unequivocal: "I *shall be* who I *shall be.*" According to Rabbi Lawrence Kushner, "Here is a Name (and a God), who is neither completed nor finished. This God is literally *not yet.*"[10] The crisis in the creation process was that the dynamic operations intrinsic to God's perfection were flawed. God's perfection entails imperfection. God needs a future to achieve completeness; hence God's reply to Moses, which admits as much. The perfection of God's being ("I *am*") is still in the process of becoming ("I *shall be*") whatever it is. Moreover, as Luria insists, God needs our assistance to achieve this goal. According to Rabbi Marc-Alain Quaknin, as human beings accept the responsibility of offering this assistance, their "ethic is no longer that of perfection but of perfectability."[11] Not being God, that is the best we can do for the One who, with an awesome interruption, acknowledged our existence in the beginning. We return the favor by heeding God's call for help. Rabbi Abraham Heschel's way of phrasing the last point is noteworthy: "All of human history as described in the Bible may be summarized in one phrase: *God is in search of man.*"[12]

The kabbalistic tradition teaches that the search is in part accomplished when human beings are successful in "raising holy sparks." The achievement is exhibited when we act in ways that are instructive for helping others to understand what it takes to be wise, virtuous, wholehearted, a doer of good deeds. The list could go on. Raising holy sparks heeds the ethic of perfectibility. God has a way of cultivating this ethic. It was evident "in the beginning" and before that, too: the use of interruption. The kabbalistic tradition returns us to the story of Adam and Eve to explain why and how God works this way. This time, however, the serpent who initiated the couple's problems is included in the story.

With its classic interpretation of the tale, Christianity makes clear that it is wise to know the Devil's work. In the kabbalistic tradition, however, the serpent means more than that. The kabbalistic teaching is that Satan is not merely the lowly and horrible creature that rules the underworld but is instead "the force of fragmentation" or interruption that operates in the physical universe as a crucial element required for creation. According to Rabbi Cooper, this does not mean, however, "that the splintering force of Satan is separate from the unity of God, but, paradoxically, that it is contained within the oneness of the Divine." Whenever the force of fragmentation (the serpent's interrupting bite) makes itself known in our lives by way of some conflict or crisis, we are given the chance to develop "messianic consciousness" and thus an awesome sense of what life is all about. "Without the serpent," writes Cooper, "without the energizing of creation, we would never have the opportunity to follow a path returning us to our Divine Source."[13] This path takes form and progresses as we raise holy sparks. The Judaic tradition emphasizes how engaging in argumentation and debate about the true meaning of God's Word is a fundamental way of performing this divine act. These communicative practices require some degree of rhetorical competence and, if the truth be told, an appreciation of the perfectionist impulse of language.[14]

The cosmological myth of the force of fragmentation parallels in several ways what I said earlier about the interruptive nature of God's command regarding perfection. The force of fragmentation operates as an interruption of our everyday existence; it opens us to matters that have yet to be properly understood; it calls us into question; it calls for action that can raise holy sparks and thereby acknowledge God; it thereby grants us the opportunity to perfect our rhetorical competence and our appreciation of the perfectionist impulse of language. God wants us to seek the truth and to do the good. Serving God in this way is emotionally satisfying and uplifting, especially if we can develop messianic consciousness. We acknowledge God, and God acknowledges us. The reciprocal relationship is the basis of the formation of human dignity.

Importantly, the myth of the force of fragmentation would also have us think differently about interruption: Its workings originate before the beginning of creation, when God withdraws "from Itself into Itself" so to make room for the creation. The dynamics of interruption are also contained in "the unity of the Divine." I noted earlier that God is a rhetorician. Now it can also be said that God is an interruption. Owing to this feature of its existence, God admits that Its perfection is a question yet to be answered. God is completely incomplete, perfectly imperfect. God is in the process of becoming what God is. To "walk before [God] and be thou perfect" is to involve ourselves in this process whereby we accept the responsibility of helping God achieve perfection. Whether you are or are not a believer, the dynamics at work here are intriguing. Think of it this way: If you were a god and wanted to create a fundamental dynamic of human existence that would ensure that sooner or later, especially in crises, people would have occasion to give some thought to the possibility of your demanding but still loving presence, I think it is fair to say that the existential dynamic of our interruptive nature would be a rather marvelous invention. Human existence is so structured that it continually calls us into question, thereby challenging us to assume the ethical burden of our freedom of choice. Your inventive act of creation is rhetorical: the first-ever use of an interruptive dynamic to encourage open-mindedness and responsible thought and action. The Holy Scriptures put this ontological and rhetorical happening into words and narratives: "Where art thou?," "Here I am!" Your act of rhetorical competence encouraged the writing of the most widely read book in the history of humankind. Indeed, the Bible nurtures metaphysical creatures longing for completeness, perfection, in you (whoever or whatever you are). You give and receive the life-giving gift of acknowledgment. You have what you wanted all along. Openness toward others is your most favored way of being. A rule of reciprocity takes form: acknowledgment.

Acknowledgment is a gift that ought to be shared. Indeed, what would life be like if no one acknowledged your existence? The power and influence of religion stands and falls on the phenomenon of acknowledgment and people's belief that when no one else in the world will help them with their pain and sorrow, they can always turn to something higher to receive this life-giving gift. Acknowledgment is a matter of health—and more. Remember that the enactment of the phenomenon as an interruption is first used by God "in the beginning." Without acknowledgment, nothing exists. Without acknowledgment, God has nothing to do. Without acknowledgment, God does not make sense. Without acknowledgment, God is a vacuous concept.

We are at a point in my story that is especially significant. God tells us that we were created in God's image (Genesis 1:27). We have an empirically based vision of what to some extent this image is. Recall what I said in the introduction about the interruption that we are. This interruption shows itself in the primordial and continual way that the future orientation of our spatial-temporal existence opens us to its ever-present dimension of uncertainty, thereby calling into question (interrupting) our self-assured beliefs that what we know about the everyday ways and means of life is correct. Like God, we are an interruption. Like God, the interruption that we are is open-ended, future-oriented, and thus always confronting itself with the uncertainty of what is not yet here and now in its existence. Like God, our interruptive nature is perfectly structured to call into question its perfection, what exactly it is. Like God, our interruptive nature finds itself in a process where what will be is necessarily a concern. Like God, our interruptive nature shows itself to be completely incomplete, perfectly imperfect. Our interruptive nature grants us an image of what God is going through as God waits for us to raise holy sparks. We are encouraged to assume the task as we deal with those situations that arise when interruptions interrupt our everyday existence and expose us to the interruption that we are. In such situations it may be necessary to demonstrate our rhetorical competence for the purpose of telling the truth about the matters at hand. Putting to use the perfectionist impulse of language thus becomes a necessity. God, the rhetorician, demands nothing less. The moral integrity and health of the lived body are on the line. So, too, human dignity.

The Judean-Christian tradition takes us back to the beginnings of interruption. There is much to consider with what this tradition has to say about this most creative event. Related phenomena include the essence of questions, acknowledgment, the creation of openings, perfection, wholeheartedness (the emotional capacity of the lived body), the perfectionist impulse of language, truth, the art of rhetoric, eloquence, eugenics, holy sparks, argumentation and debate, respect, goodness (living a good life), human dignity, moral integrity, and others as well. These phenomena will continue to warrant attention as my story develops. There are virtues listed here that are particularly important for my purposes. In attending now to what science has to say about the beginnings of interruption, the story has to change a bit.

Science

What science tells us about the beginnings and consequences of interruption turns religion on its head. Science doesn't deny the existence of the phenomena I have noted; it just refuses to believe that we need God to explain their presence. God is not our creator. Rather, we created God by way of the rhetorical construction of a narrative that enables us to deal in a meaningful manner with the interruption that we are and our mental and behavioral reactions to it. So, for example, it feels good to imagine a god that once promised us that one day we could "walk before [whatever it is] and be thou perfect." Human beings love the thought. We are creatures who yearn for completeness in our lives. That's evolution, nothing more, although the narrative of science is not free of dissent on this matter. There are more than a few remarkable scientists who are also strong believers in God's holy presence.[15]

A major objective of the eighteenth-century philosopher and empiricist David Hume was to discredit the doctrines and dogmas of orthodox religious belief; they are based on myth and speculation rather than on verifiable evidence. Hume did admit, however, that "Wherever I see order, I infer from experience that *there,* there hath been design and contrivance. And the same principle which leads me into this inference, when I contemplate a building, regular and beautiful in its whole frame and structure; the same principle obliges me to infer an infinitely perfect architect, from the infinite art and contrivance which is displayed in the whole fabric of the Universe."[16] Hume offers here a version of Intelligent Design theory, which maintains that physical and biological systems observed in the universe result chiefly from purposeful design by an intelligent being rather than from chance and other undirected natural processes. I suspect that supporters of the theory would point to the interruption that we are as an illustration of their worldview.[17]

The building Hume refers to is an example of how human beings have a desire for completeness in their lives—an admirable passion for "perfection."

This passion plays a fundamental role in our social and political existence as we attempt to sustain and advance the progress we have achieved in the struggle to survive, understand the world, be better persons, and live the good life. Although he does not say so, efforts to create things that are "regular and beautiful in [their] whole frame and structure" would qualify as attempts to raise holy sparks and cultivate perfect wisdom. Hume also emphasizes, however, that, in the great scheme of things, such efforts, no matter how successful they may be, are humbling to the point of embarrassment: "Man falls much more short of perfect wisdom, and even of his own ideas of perfect wisdom, than animals do of man; yet the latter difference is so considerable, that nothing but a comparison with the former can make it appear of little moment."[18] And Hume's skepticism goes even further. When considering the debate over the morality of suicide and how "God-fearing" souls used their ultimate understanding of perfection to decry the sinfulness of this final act, Hume claims that "the life of a man is of no greater importance to the universe than that of an oyster."[19] An empirical orientation toward the world may encourage people to engage in metaphysical speculation, but empiricism is steadfast in its commitment to sticking to the tangible physical data that can be measured with as much precision as possible. Empiricism seeks perfection and leaves it at that. Acquiring knowledge of sensible reality is in and of itself rewarding.

Hume's inference regarding a "perfect architect" who *may* have designed "the whole fabric of the universe" is not incommensurate with his unflattering view of "the life of man." Science supports this view with what it tells us about the occurrence of an interruption that marked the beginning of the cosmos: the big bang, that primordial explosion and opening of a highly compact universe that originated approximately 13.7 billion years ago and that is at least 150 billion light-years across and growing.[20] Light travels 186,000 miles per second, so we are talking about quite a big place here. Think about it: Calculate the number of seconds there are in a year. Multiply that by 186,000. Now multiply that figure by 13.7 billion. And keep in mind that the cosmos is still expanding. So, yes, given the numbers, our significance in the universe is quite insignificant. Oysters have company. Carefully calculated numbers suggest as much. Numbers are science's version of the perfectionist function of language.

Yet, science points to another interruption that elevates our status in the great scheme of things. The cosmologist and astrophysicist Martin Rees directs us toward this interruption when he notes: "Our universe sprouted from an initial event, the 'big bang' or 'fireball.' It expanded and cooked; the intricate pattern of stars and galaxies we see around us emerged thousands of millions of years later; on at least one planet around at least one star, atoms have assembled into creatures complex enough to ponder how they evolved."[21] To ponder some object, topic, or set of circumstances requires a certain act of consciousness, one that is willing and able to interrupt the daily routinized ways of seeing and thinking about one's environment and become open and remain attentive to what something is. With the evolutionary development of this particular cognitive capacity and the related capacity to symbolize and thereby generate a mutual understanding of reality, human beings assumed a fundamental role in the event of the universe becoming aware of itself to some extent. Owing to their interruptive ability to ponder, human beings open a place in space and time where, as philosophers often put it, "Being" itself is given a chance to be acknowledged and appreciated. As noted, the kabbalistic tradition associates this place (*makom*) with the existence of the lived body and its heartfelt ability to experience God's presence in the world. The only chance we have to know anything of reality is to be open to it. The ability to ponder is a talent that, as far as I know, oysters don't have. Acknowledgment is a privilege of humankind.

Here is Rees pondering how the results of science's mathematical calculations of the beginnings of our solar system within the ever-expanding cosmos require a radical change in our common way of appreciating space and time: "Suppose America had existed forever, and you were walking across it, starting on the East Coast when the Earth formed, and ending up in California when the Sun was about to die. To make this journey, you'd have to take *one step every two thousand years.* A mere three or four steps would represent all recorded history. . . . Our sun is less than halfway [4.5 billion years] through its life; we are still near the 'simple beginning' of the evolutionary story."[22] With the science of cosmology to guide our pondering, we must realize that from "the beginning" to the sixth day, when God created and acknowledged "man," marks a period of billions of years. The precision of mathematical calculations enables us to appreciate, for example, the wrongheadedness of religious myth. The Judean-Christian tradition offers a narrative that is nonsense. The Nobel Prize–winning physicist and atheist Steven Weinberg puts it this way: "One of the great achievements of science has been, if not to make it impossible for intelligent people to be religious, then at least to make it possible for them not to be religious. We should not retreat from this accomplishment."[23] The dignity of science demands as much.

Everyday interruptions can incite the interruptive workings of pondering. For example, I am going through the mindless routines of getting ready to go to work. I hear a story on the radio about some guy going into a high school and shooting and killing fifteen students. The news stops me dead in my tracks and gives me pause for thought. "How can people be so sick? How are these kids' parents going to survive this horror?" I sit down and ponder some more. I will be late for work. I remain seated, pondering, until I cannot take it anymore. Pondering is not always pleasant. Still, it serves a valuable purpose. We need to be open to the world so that, for example, we can advance our understanding of matters of importance and think about what needs to be done to improve our lives and the lives of others. Sometimes the interruption that sets off the interruptive workings of pondering can just come from inside one's own head. I'm lying in bed, relaxed, nothing on my mind, all my work done for the day. Peacefulness. Solitude. I'm really getting into it. It's rare, but it happens. And then, from out of nowhere, or so it seems, an idea for a research project pops into my head. Pondering begins. I stay open to the idea. I am no longer relaxing. But I'm excited. It feels good. I jump out of bed, run to the computer, and start making notes. I'm still pondering. What if the idea is not as good as I first thought it was? Pondering continues. Stay open! Stay open! Keep the interruption going. The significance of the lived body's presence in the universe is demonstrating itself, if only with an N of 1.

Scientists are in the business of pondering. Their disciplined empirical outlook demands nothing less. They must stay open to their object of investigation if they are to be true to the object's truth, to how it is disclosing itself to witnesses. The Nobel Prize–winning physicist Richard Feynman has this obligation in mind when he emphasizes how in science "openness to possibility is an opportunity. Doubt and discussion are essential to progress."[24] The conscientious scientist is forever engaged in discovery, creating theory, testing it out, and inviting others to show that what he or she has accomplished is wrong or, at best, basically insignificant. This procedure is often painful: It hurts to have one's work called into question. But that is the greatness of science; that is how it ensures that pondering will be sustained in the quest for truth. Science heads in the direction of proving the truth by designing research that is intended to interrupt what is presently claimed to be the truth. To quote Weinberg, "the decision to explore the world as it is shown to us by reason and experiment is a moral one, not a scientific one."[25] Situated in a world of know-how, the morality of science is advanced by its drive for perfection.

This is what it took to discover the interruption of the big bang. No pondering, no big bang as far as we know. Highly sophisticated research and mathematical theory in cosmology and astrophysics allow scientists to comprehend what was going on with the big bang from approximately one ten-billionth of a second after it took place. The instant before this grand opening happened, however, is another story. That story must be told as science adheres to a fundamental ethic that guides its much-valued goal of being objective: pondering and openmindedness. This state of mind invites as yet noticeable aspects of reality to interrupt what was thought to be the case. Science lives and breathes interruption.

Coming to know that the big bang happened and how it happened is a moral endeavor. Before the big bang blasted into being everything in the universe, there may have existed what cosmologists term a "singularity," which is the nearest thing that science has found to a supernatural agent. At a singularity, so the theory goes, one finds a state of infinite temperature, density, and energy condensed into a point the size of an infinitesimal speck of dust; here, space-time as we know it does not exist. A singularity exists outside space-time, or what cosmologists sometimes describe as a state of "nothingness." Before the big bang there was something that was nothing, a presence of absence from which emerged all the material of the universe that will ever exist. The big bang was not an explosion in space but an explosion of all measurable (timely) space, an explosion whose echo is still detectable as long-wavelength radiation or what is also called the cosmic microwave background. This explosion began in the beginning but is not itself the beginning. Rather, it is an effect of something, perhaps a singularity that came *before* it, out of nothing and nowhere.

Speculation regarding "the before" of the big bang is based on science's mathematical ability to extrapolate from what is known about the observable universe and predict what was going on in a state of nothingness and nowhere. So, for example, there is Alan Guth's theory of cosmic inflation, from the early 1980s, which explains how our universe has been expanding since the big bang. This theory, which is built into the standard quantum theory of elementary particles, grants the possibility that the phenomenon of inflation was happening prior to the big bang. The inflation may be due to the presence of "dark energy." Dark energy is neither atomic nor visible, which is to say that it is not composed of quarks and electrons. This energy, which defines approximately 70 percent of the density of our present day cosmos, is in conflict with gravity: The presence of regular matter causes the expansion ratio of the universe to slow down, while dark energy speeds it up. In a heuristic sense, then, dark energy acts as if it is a repulsive force, and just before the big bang occurred the repulsion inflated exponentially, instigating an interruption of momentous proportion. Out of a location of nothingness and nowhere (a "space" that is dramatically otherwise than everyday space) came the existence of the universe. The more space grew, the more repulsion and inflation transpired. The universe is expanding. There are currently more than 100 billion galaxies in the observable universe. The most distant of these galaxies are receding from us at a velocity approaching the speed of light; other universes are emerging in the process.[26]

Other universes! According to the theory of cosmic inflation, our universe is not the only universe in the entire cosmos, and singularities need not have been necessary for the event to happen. Rather, universes are part of an "eternal inflation" process that has been enduring since before the beginning of what we understand to be time. Moments of cosmic inflation give rise perhaps to big bangs that evolve into separate universes. Our universe is but a minuscule part of a much larger, ever-inflating cosmic order or "multiverse" containing perhaps billions of other universes with their own billions of galaxies.[27] Speaking metaphorically, science suggests that the universe is but a "bubble" emerging from the ocean's ebb and flow, an infinitely brief interruption of a process that continues as the interruption begins another evolving universe. What is the cause of this interruption? At the present time, science is unable to answer the question. What cosmologists term "God-of-the-gaps" thinking—that is, giving God credit for what we do not know—is not allowed when doing rigorous scientific research. The theoretical physicist Paul Davies tells us why: "Our ignorance of the origin of life leaves plenty of scope for divine explanation, but that is a purely negative attitude, invoking 'the God-of-the-gaps' only to risk retreat at a later date in the face of scientific advances." Hence, "to invoke God as a blanket explanation of the unexplained is to invite eventual falsification, and make God the friend of ignorance. If God is to be found, it must surely be through what we discover about the world not what we fail to discover."[28] Such discoveries are, to be sure, forms of interruption that change our consciousness of the world. For, indeed, consciousness dawns with the second experience, with an interruption of taken-for-granted behavior that discloses what such behavior hides with its familiarity and singular mind-set.

In his discussion of the wonders of evolution, the scientist and theologian Pierre Teilhard de Chardin speaks of this interruptive moment of consciousness. It is an awareness of the world that had the cognitive and reflective capacity to turn its attention back to itself, interrupting its one-way intention toward the world to become self-conscious. The consequences of this act, maintains Chardin, "are immense, visible as clearly in nature as any of the facts recorded by physics or astronomy": "The being who is the object of his own reflection . . . becomes in a flash able to raise himself into a new sphere. In reality, another world is born. Abstraction, logic, reasoned choice and inventions, mathematics, art, calculation of space and time, anxieties and dreams of love—all these activities of *inner life* are nothing else than the effervescence of the newly-formed centre as it explodes onto itself." Chardin describes this explosion of consciousness as a "discontinuity in continuity," an immensely important interruption of the process of evolution, a moment when the lived body is born and "cerebral perfectioning" must be cultivated to ensure the "progress" of humankind.[29]

One might say that the interruption that incites the dawning of consciousness is its own big bang, its own opening of a space and time where amazing and horrible things can happen. Progress is associated with the first of these options. The physician Lewis Thomas addresses this notion of progress when explaining "the greatest single achievement of nature today": "the invention of the molecule of DNA." He writes: "We have had it from the very beginning, built into the first cell to emerge, membranes and all, somewhere in the soupy water of the cooling planet three thousand million years or so ago. All of today's DNA, strung through all the cells of the earth, is simply an extension and elaboration of that first molecule. In a fundamental sense we cannot claim to have made progress, since the method used for growth and replication is essentially unchanged."[30]

Thomas, however, would still have us appreciate the importance of the term, even though "it is out of fashion today to talk of progress in evolution if you use that word to mean anything like improvement, implying some sort of value judgment beyond the reach of science." Thomas admits that he "cannot think of a better term to describe what has happened," and with remarkable eloquence he makes his point: "After all, to have come all the way from a system of life possessing only one kind of primitive microbial cell, living out colorless lives in hummocks of algal mats, to what we see around us today—the City of Paris, the State of Iowa, Cambridge University, Woods Hole, the succession of travertine-lined waterfall and lakes like flights of great stairs in Yugoslavia's Plitvice, the horse chestnut tree in my backyard, and the columns of neurons arranged in modules in the cerebral cortex of vertebrates—has to represent improvement. We have come a long way on that old molecule."[31]

Importantly, however, Thomas would have us realize that such progress presupposes "the real marvel of DNA": "its capacity to blunder slightly," to have its life sustained with the help of mutations that interrupt its past and present status. "Without this special attribute, we would still be anaerobic bacteria and there would be no music," quips Thomas. "Viewed individually, one by one, each of the mutations that have brought us along represent a random, totally spontaneous accident, but it is no accident at all that mutations occur; the molecule of DNA was ordained from the beginning to make small mistakes."[32]

Mistakes are interruptions in what would otherwise be the developing sequence of a thought or action intended to reach a specific goal or endpoint. Thomas admits that we "prefer sticking to the point, and insuring ourselves against chance. But there it is: we are here by the purest of chance, and by mistake at that. Somewhere along the line, nucleotides were edged apart to let new ones in; maybe viruses moved in, carrying along bits of other, foreign genomes; radiation from the sun or from outer space caused tiny cracks in the molecule, and humanity was conceived." The lesson is clear: Life as we know it scientifically is impossible without the force of interruption being at work. Thomas's final way of making the point is noteworthy: "[I]f you have a mechanism designed to keep changing the ways of living, and if all the new forms have to fit together as they plainly do, and if every improvised new gene representing an embellishment in an individual is likely to be selected for the species, and if you have enough time, maybe the system is simply bound to develop brains sooner or later, and awareness."[33]

We are the product of interruptions. Recall that Thomas speaks of being "ordained" with this interruptive nature. I do not interpret his use of this religiously tinged word as indicating anything more than a point of origin, perhaps a force—a "mechanism," as he notes—that has always been at work with its interruptive dynamic. Thomas tells us that science teaches us to be respectful of a phenomenon whose history is traceable only to this point, thus coming to us from we know not where, and that enacts a force that is life-giving. Evolution has a progressive impulse for improvement, at least now that it has reached the stage of human beings, with their ability to ponder the interruption that we are. The moral nature of science suggests as much. For Chardin, this impulse grants hope that a convergence with the Divine is possible. Science, too, cherishes this hope. But it is evolution, not God, that validates the possibility that a more perfect world is yet to come. In the beginning was an interruption. One need not go any further than the big bang and the theory of eternal inflation to come to terms with the source of the impulse that materialized into humanity. And this being the case, science turns religion on its head.

Yes, the interruption that we are is a product of our future-oriented existence exposing us to uncertainty. This temporal orientation is the result of a 13.7-billion-year-old interrupting explosion that directed and is still directing the cosmos toward the uncertainty of the unknown, otherwise called the openness of the future. Confronting the uncertainty of existence is a well-known cause of anxiety. A primary way that human beings deal with the ill and sometimes terrifying effects of this emotion is by creating narratives that help us cope with uncertainty as they provide meaningful and purposeful direction in our lives. The most famous of these narratives is religion, with its perfectionist and moral worldview. Science presents us with another narrative that also admits such a worldview. This narrative is famous, too, but for a much different reason: It avoids at all costs the metaphysical route of religion. The beginning interruption was not a holy event but only a chance occurrence. God didn't create us. We, being the interruption that we are, created God. Science accepts that we are an interruption, that the health of the lived body is a matter of unquestionable importance, and that the rhetorical construction of narratives assists in our structuring of existence. These phenomena are effects of a cause that never said "Let there be" nor asked "Where art thou?" Being exposed to the interruption that we are can lead to the production of all kinds of revered and repulsive thoughts and behaviors: hence the various related topics introduced when discussing religion. But it is simply the case that these thoughts and behaviors are ways in which the progressive impulse of evolution materialized into humanity. And perhaps there is more to come in the life of this impulse.

The theoretical physicist Lee Smolin believes so. What he suggests is stunning. He ponders: The future does not yet exist and is therefore open. We can reasonably infer some predictions, but we cannot predict the future completely. Indeed, the future can produce phenomena that are genuinely novel, in the sense that no knowledge of the past could have anticipated them. Nothing transcends time, not even the laws of nature. Laws are not timeless. Like everything else, they are features of the present, and they can evolve over time.[34] You might say to this: "Impossible. We are talking about the fundamental laws of nature. They are 13.7 billion years old." Yes, but the cosmos is still expanding and thus so is the uncertainty of the future; 13.7 billion years comes nowhere close to saying it all. If Smolin is right, science will have a lot of pondering to do. Its world of know-how and attending perfectionist and moral narrative will come face to face with the interruption that we are, if it is still around. For the time being, however, the interruption that we are and its perfective function remain essential features of human existence. Science will welcome you into its world of know-how and invite you to contribute to its narrative about the origins and destiny of interruption, unless what you have to say supports the argument of Intelligent Design. God-of-the-gaps thinking insults the moral imperative of science. The interruption that we are is a given. Let it be.

Science, however, does not put an end to assessments of the interruption that we are. Be they religious or not, these assessments allow for a more refined understanding of the interruption than has been offered so far. In telling a story about this interruption, I welcome their input. The three that I find most informative are those of Søren Kierkegaard, Martin Heidegger, and Emmanuel Levinas. Kierkegaard brings religion back on the scene. Although not a scientist, Heidegger avoids God-of-the-gaps thinking. Levinas finds a way to accommodate both of these approaches. Kierkegaard and Heidegger focus their attention on the existence of the self. Levinas focuses his attention on the existence of the other. I find problems with all three assessments. Nevertheless, what they have to offer to a story about the interruption that we are is instructive.

CHAPTER 2

Existence and the Self

"No one dares to be himself; everyone is hiding in 'togetherness'."

Søren Kierkegaard, *Provocations*

....

"Selfhood is to be discerned existentially only in one's authentic potentiality-for-Being-one's Self."

Martin Heidegger, *Being and Time*

....

In his book, *Our Improbable Universe,* the physicist Michael Murray feels compelled to think about the source of evolution's progressive impulse. The big bang, for sure. But Murray does not dismiss the possibility that "a creator" was behind the scenes. So he wonders:

> Was this improbable and incredible process [of evolution] the result of a trillion billion throws of the universe-creating dice? Or was it all designed from the start in such a clever way that the subsequent evolutionary developments were, in a general sense, inevitable? . . . What might the motivation to create have been? Why didn't the artist sign the canvas? Is there a signature? . . . What can we know about the creator itself? If the universe was created, then the creator has to be a fantastic artist/engineer/philosopher/everything. . . . The creator must have been fascinated with the task and derived satisfaction from the results. How could a creator keep it a secret? Wouldn't a signature on the canvas be compulsory? Why would a creator resist the temptation to sign?[1]

Søren Kierkegaard

Kierkegaard's writings lead one to believe that the interruption that we are is the Creator's signature on the canvas. Kierkegaard phrases it this way: "The essential sermon is one's own existence."[2] He thus tells us that in order to form an authentic understanding of God, "One must first learn to know oneself before knowing anything else. . . . Only when the person has inwardly understood *himself,* and then sees the way forward on his path, does his life acquire repose and meaning."[3] Kierkegaard combines these two claims when he notes: "Existence constitutes the highest interest of the existing individual, and his interest in his existence constitutes his reality."[4]

Quotations such as these make clear Kierkegaard's unwavering belief that God's signature lies no further way than one's own existence. The structure and function of existence teach us how to think and act such that we become genuinely attuned to God's presence. Kierkegaard takes exception to those who display a passive allegiance to the institutionalized habits of Christian doctrine because such allegiance promotes only a "dead calm" wherein people no longer struggle to become Christians but allow themselves to be lulled into an inauthentic state of "easiness." This state of being, where questions, actions, and personal decisions are drowned in the calm of Christian dogma, is for Kierkegaard a crisis. To counter this crisis, Kierkegaard chooses to "create difficulties" against Christendom; for he believes that "*it is easier to become a Christian when I am not a Christian than to become a Christian when I am one.*"[5] Christendom is a world of know-how whose narrative disables its inhabitants from coming to know the truth of God's ways. Kierkegaard is a living interruption of this narrative. He wants Christians to hear and take seriously the essential sermon of existence. If they are to become authentic in their faith, they have to come face to face with the interruption that we are.

Kierkegaard is convinced that his self-appointed task to move people beyond the "rut" of Christendom is justified. He states, "For when it comes to a crisis, the carriage sticks fast and cannot be moved, or threatens to turn over in the ruts, the driver will use the whip, not from cruelty, but convinced that it will help the horses, and only mollycoddles hesitate to strike."[6] Kierkegaard does not hesitate to strike. The most truthful education we receive about God comes not from sermons aligned with Christian dogma but rather from the empirical ground of the self's existence, which is its own demonstration. The constantly occurring lived experience of human being requires no manner of abstract thought to prove its presence. *Cogito ergo sum?* No, the "I am" must always come first. Thought presupposes existence; it is but a way of existing. Hence, if the question of what it means to exist is to be answered in an experientially adequate and authentic fashion, then one must return to his or her own concrete existence as it is actually being lived and experienced so to witness and describe the demonstration at hand.

Kierkegaard emphasizes how the lived body's finitude exhibits a dialectical relationship with infinity: the ever-present uncertainty of the future. Human existence is always caught up in "the process of becoming" what is not yet in a lived body's life. I noted in the Introduction that Kierkegaard employs an oxymoron to describe this dialectic of human existence: "Objective uncertainty." An oxymoron is a rhetorical figure (Gk. "a witty, paradoxical saying") employed for effect, for stimulating the attunement of consciousness when making a point. An oxymoron is an interruption meant to conflict with common sense, give pause for thought with its contradicting nature, incite an enhanced and perfected appreciation of the matter under consideration, and thereby make a difference in our lives. It may thus be said that the essential sermon of existence, the interruption that we are, shows itself to be a rhetorical interruption. Kierkegaard emphasizes that the self's existence "preaches [this rhetorically interrupting] sermon every hour of the day and with power quite different from that of the most eloquent speaker in his most eloquent movement. To let your mouth run with eloquent babbling when such talk is the opposite of your life is in the deepest sense nonsense. You become liable to eternal judgment."[7]

Human existence speaks (preaches) God's existence: objective uncertainty. We are an oxymoron. We are an interruption. We are rhetorical beings. Eloquent babbling, however, deafens us to the sermon that is the interruption that we are. Kierkegaard associates such babbling with what he finds going on in the preaching that the institution of Christendom requires its clergy to speak during scheduled services. Eloquent babbling or "talkativeness" is also a trait of what Kierkegaard calls the "public," the "crowd," and the "herd." These terms depict the mindless conformism that habitats of everyday worlds of know-how can foster with their rules, routines, habits, linguistic practices (eloquent babbling), and standards of common sense. The novelist Vladimir Nabokov has the problem in mind when he declares that "Common sense is sense made common, so everything is comfortably cheapened by its touch."[8] Here are two examples of Kierkegaard making the point when commenting on how selves lose their authenticity as they cater to the will of the crowd and the herd: "Hence where there is a multitude, a crowd, or where decisive significance is attached to the fact that there is a multitude, there it is sure that no one is working, living, striving for the highest aim, but only for one or another early aim; since to work for the eternal decisive aim is possible only where there is one, and to be this one which all can be is to let God be the helper—the 'crowd' is the untruth . . . by reason of the fact that it renders the individual completely impenitent and irresponsible, or at least weakens his sense of responsibility by reducing it to a fraction."[9] "If you want to be loathsome to God, just run with the herd."[10]

For Kierkegaard, the only way to avoid this fearful judgment is to be instructed not by the eloquent babblings of Christian dogma but rather by the teachings of existence: how it is that we are always in the process of becoming, always being confronted by uncertainty, and thus always having to assume the ethical responsibility of making our *own* choice of how to form an authentic relationship with God. Assuming this responsibility requires that we make the best use of the perfective impulse of the interruption that we are—time and again. As the philosopher Paul Brockelman notes, "Selves are not things 'in' time, but temporal *processes* or *dynamic activities.* Selves are tensed."[11] In constructing his dialectical system of logic to suggest how the reality of existence could be captured in a final "moment" of speculative consciousness allowing for an understanding of God as "Absolute Spirit," the philosopher Georg Wilhelm Friedrich Hegel confounded the self's temporal existence by reducing it to the timeless and logical "becoming" of pure abstract thought. For the concrete, existing self, however, *time is of the essence.* To be a self is to become a self, and to become a self is to be forever caught up in the temporal and historical process of acting out one's own existence for as long as one lives. With both Hegel and this last point in mind, Kierkegaard writes: "To be finished with life before life has finished with one, is precisely not to have finished the task."[12] Immersed in his system of logic, Hegel thought he finished the task; his own existence, which is to say his self, proved otherwise. The interruption that we are is more than a system of logic.

Kierkegaard would have us say "yes" to the self, to the individual who has taken on the responsibility of his freedom to choose his destiny. Selfhood is achieved through such individualization, through the personal enactment of our freedom of choice that comes with our being open to the future, the "not yet" of a person's life, and the anxiety brought about by this openness of existence. "What is anxiety?" asks Kierkegaard. "It is the next day," the day you can die at any moment. Anxiety and the inevitability of death go hand in hand.[13] Still, selfhood remains an ever-present task, and if we are to perform this task authentically, we must assume the responsibility of enacting our freedom of choice. We must choose our way of being, or others (the crowd) will simply choose it for us. The options are as simple as they are important: either to choose or to be chosen, either to achieve integrity through resolute choice or to lose integrity through retreat from choice. Although the orderly functions of our habits of living can all too easily have us forsake and forget its presence, we cannot escape this either/or, this condition of existence. "As truly as there is a future," writes Kierkegaard, "just so truly is there an either/or."[14] In any given situation, the decision not to assume the responsibility of making choices is still to have chosen not to choose. For Kierkegaard, there is nothing more important that an individual can recognize and say "yes" to than what he or she is as a self that is always in the historical process of becoming itself through its freedom of choice. With this recognition and affirmation comes the courage of self-determination, the courage to question the conformist nature of the crowd that seeks to corrupt the self's freedom by conditioning it to think, preach, and practice only those customized habits and routines sanctioned by the crowd or the herd. Kierkegaard employs the story of Elvira in the opera *Don Juan* to illustrate this self-affirming process of authenticity—a virtue that Kierkegaard maintains is the hallmark of human dignity.[15]

Elvira had been a nun. Because of her passion for Don Juan, she abandons the cloister to live with him. However, after seducing her, Don Juan abandons Elvira. She now stands alone, left to reflect on the facticity of her existential situation. "She has lost everything—heaven when she chose the world, the world when she lost Don Juan" (193). As she reflects on her situation, she realizes her task: She must strive to give her situation a new meaning, a new narrative; she must locate an ethic to live by; she must become something more than the grieved person she now is. She thus proceeds to act by deliberating with herself; that is, she starts to speak the truth of her situation with the hope of discovering alternatives that she can choose from to direct her future.

As her soliloquy takes form, one senses that Elvira is authentic, for she speaks in terms of possibilities. Her first possibility is to give her life meaning by hating Don Juan: "I will hate him; only so can my soul find satisfaction, only so can I find rest and occupation for my thoughts. . . . This shall be my work, my task, to which I dedicate myself" (200). But in seeing this first possibility, Elvira also realizes that it was Juan's love that granted her life so much meaning. Thus, she forms another possibility directly opposed to the first possibility: "No, I will be proud that he loved me, that he was greater than the gods, and I will honor him by making myself nothing" (201–2). This second possibility in turn moves her back to her first possibility: "No, I cannot think of him; every time I remember him, every time my thought approaches the hiding place in my heart where his memory dwells, then it is as if I committed a new sin" (202).

Elvira now must declare her freedom by choosing one of the alternatives; if she is to remain authentic, she must accept the fact that her chosen course is made possible only by the alternative she did not choose. Thus, her deliberation makes her decision difficult by taking away the easy approach of seeing her situation in terms of a direct either/or perspective; that is, it is not the case that her situation consists of either the first possibility or the second possibility. The facticity of the situation demands that both possibilities exist and that both may be chosen.

In one sense, Elvira remains authentic, for she realizes the paradoxical anguish of her possibilities and she admits it: "If I could remember [Juan] with the anguish, I would not be remembering him" (202). But Elvira lacks the courage to choose, and thus the possibility for a future self activity, wherein a new narrative and ethical approach to life could become operative, is thwarted by her own mental torment. Elvira's authenticity is halted by her indecisiveness; she never succeeds in transforming her consciousness to enacted behavior, her theoretical possibilities to praxis. The result is that she becomes a victim of her own anguish. As Kierkegaard puts it: "she considers over and over again, she seizes every way out, and yet she finds none, and so she can never grieve connectically and roundly, because she always seeks to discover how she ought to grieve"

(200). Becoming and remaining an authentic self is an arduous task. Kierkegaard tells us that "If there were no eternal consciousness in a man, if at the bottom of everything there were only a wild ferment, a power that twisting in dark passions produced everything great or inconsequential; if an unfathomable, insatiable emptiness lay hid beneath everything, what would life be but despair?"[16] His words could be an epitaph for Elvira. He also offers an insight that could have been instructive as she languishes staring directly at the interruption that we are: "Learning to know dread [anxiety] is an adventure which every man has to affront if he would not go to perdition either by not having known dread or by sinking under it. He therefore who has learned rightly to be in dread has learned the most important thing."[17] The lesson speaks to the virtue of being a person of dignity. If Kierkegaard were alive today, imagine his reaction were he to read the one-time tag line for the antidepressant Paxil on the GlaxoSmithKline Web site: "Relieve the anxiety, and reveal the person."[18]

Anxiety was Kierkegaard's way of being. His books were not well received by the press. His looks were unsightly. He was ridiculed as a cripple because of his hunchback. He broke off his engagement to his much-loved Regina Olsen as he made the choice for his brand of Christianity. He found no reprieve in a world of know-how, given his distaste for its conformist ways of life. Imagine what your life would be like if you had no world of know-how to lend some structure and order to your everyday existence. The confusion would be discomforting and maddening. The loneliness would be heartbreaking and depressing. Moreover, loneliness is associated with undermining learning and memory, causing intense episodes of fear and anxiety, raising levels of stress, guilt, sin, and increasing the risk of suicide.[19] These are not healthy ways to exist. Kierkegaard admits as much throughout his writings, especially those works whose titles and contents are far from inviting to contented members of the crowd: *Fear and Trembling, The Concept of Dread, The Sickness unto Death.* Yet, with respect to the world of know-how sustained by the ways and means of Christendom, Kierkegaard remains steadfast in standing face to face with the interruption that we are. Christendom's world of know-how, its crowd, and the narrative that goes with it must be called into question, no matter how much anxiety comes to the fore.

Reading Kierkegaard's critique of Christendom reminds me of the work of the contemporary philosopher Jacques Derrida and his commitment to "deconstructive" criticism. Derrida reads and interprets texts for the purpose of disclosing any of their "reified and unthinking dogmas." Deconstruction, writes Derrida, "is not *neutral.* It *intervenes*": through its "unorthodox" reading of writings, it seeks to show and tell others that there is necessarily more meaning to texts than meets the eye, especially the eye of the self that knows only how to read and interpret in conformity with "institutionalized critical methods."

Moreover, in performing this act of intervention, deconstruction offers itself to others as a way of helping them to realize that "Every culture needs an element of self-interrogation and of distance from itself, if it is to transform itself, if it is to become something different, something other and more than what it presently is under the "official political codes governing reality."[20] Indeed, Derrida tells us that the "principle theme" of deconstruction is the "destabilization" characterizing the "intertextuality" of systems of meaning. Furthermore, Derrida equates his project of deconstruction with this destabilization, which he defines as "the true source of anxiety" haunting those "conservatives" who seek only the stability of their own meaning systems or worlds of know-how.[21] You can't get more Kierkegaardian than that, at least when deconstruction's intended object of criticism is the crowd's gross misunderstanding of Christianity.

Deconstruction is content to leave people in that state of anxiety, face to face with the interruption that we are, since this procedure of criticism is not in the business of supplying productive and perfective narratives that can abide by the impulse of our interruptive nature to regain some sanctuary in a world of know-how. Kierkegaard choose to live his life at the depths of existence. He survived because he could construct a rhetorical narrative that, although it kept him in his place of choice, granted him a way of living a meaningful and dignified life—a good life—that enabled him to have faith in God and to stay away from the crowd. "Truth is subjectivity," claims Kierkegaard.[22] The claim lies at the heart of his philosophy. Truth is what the individual accepts passionately as an understanding of how life ought to be lived in accordance not with some objective determination of reality but rather with the wisdom and judgment acquired through personal experience of the burdens and benefits of existence. An illustration of what Kierkegaard is claiming is found in the emotionally intense vision of suffering that Picasso was able to disclose in his 1937 paintings *Guernica* and *Head of a Horse*. These paintings display Picasso's early cubist style of composition. The figures in the paintings are disjointed and chaotic in form rather than being picture-like representations. This Cubist style of presentation interrupts standards of common sense, thus requiring viewers to work with rather than just glance at the paintings in order to figure out and appreciate what is going on in front of the viewers' eyes.

The paintings are displays of truth, displays that, in their own way, are as reasonable and rational as the assertion "Two times two makes four." Unlike the later objective assertion, which need function only on an intellectual level for its content to be apprehended, Picasso's displays are subjective and function first and foremost on an existential level. His paintings project a protest against the brutality of fascism in particular and modern war in general; at the same time, they project the real suffering that he was experiencing and living as he visualized the pain of creatures under attack and being destroyed. The paintings are not what Picasso thinks but what he *is*, passionately; they express a subjectivity, an existential truth. Kierkegaard's claim that "truth is subjectivity" captures what is going on here. Picasso's existential truth cries out for others to appropriate it and thus make it their own. Without this act of appropriation, Picasso's truth can go no further than Picasso. Others must realize it and integrate it into their modes of existence as a directive for what must not be done to human beings and defenseless creatures. If a truth is to live on as something more than an intellectual topic, it must become subjective; it must be forever vitalized by the passion of a self. Without this passion, truth is, at best, sterile; at worst, it is dead.

In Kierkegaard's terms, the paintings are examples of the "art of communication" dedicated to "taking away" or "luring something away from someone."[23] Kierkegaard praises the "difficulty" that such art poses for viewers because it opens them to possibilities of seeing the world in ways that are different from and perhaps more insightful than those they have been conditioned to accept by the crowd. The art's function is aligned with the truth of existence: The self is open to the uncertainty of the future and thus is always in the process of becoming its possibilities. Following Kierkegaard, one can also say that the paintings' art of communication subscribes to the dialectical nature of Socratic dialogue, whereby Socrates employs maieutic artistry to draw out from his interlocutors their supposed knowledge of some topic. Recall that dialogue operates as an interruption, as does Kierkegaard and the objective uncertainty that guides his faith in the glory of God. Kierkegaard offers the following analogy to clarify how the art of communication works: "When a man has his mouth so full of food that he is prevented from eating, and is like to starve in consequence, does giving him food consist in stuffing still more of it in his mouth, or does it consist it taking some of it away, so that he can begin to eat? And so also when a man has much knowledge, and his knowledge has little or no significance for him, does a rational communication consist in giving him more knowledge, even supposing that he is loud in his insistence that this is what he needs, or does it not rather consist in taking some of it away?"[24]

The art of communication favored by Kierkegaard functions as an interruption that exposes a person to the interruption that we are. Faced with the essential sermon offered by this fundamental interruption, the person must assume the responsibility of being a self that is open to the possibility that its knowledge of the world is deficient and in need of more enlightened wisdom. In short, what Kierkegaard terms "the secret" of the art of communication "consists precisely in emancipating the recipient, and that for this reason [the speaker] must not communicate himself directly; aye, that it is even irreligious to do so."[25] Here is an example of Kierkegaard offering emancipatory discourse on the nature of the self: "Man is a spirit. But what is a spirit? Spirit is the self. But what is the self? The self is a relation which relates itself to its own self, or it is that in the relation [which accounts for it] that the relation relates itself to its own self; the self is not the relation but [consists in the fact] that the relation relates itself to its own self. . . . Such a relation which relates itself to its own self (that is to say, a self) must either have constituted itself or have been constituted by another."[26]

The comedian Woody Allen reports reading this passage when he was convalescing from an illness and had nothing else to do but glance over some books on philosophy. Responding specifically to the definition of the self contained in the passage, Allen offers this sarcastic and humorous response: "The concept brought tears to my eyes. My word, I thought, to be that clever! (I'm a man who has trouble writing two meaningful sentences on 'My Day at the Zoo.') True, the passage was totally incomprehensible to me, but what of it as long as Kierkegaard was having fun?"[27]

Kierkegaard was known for wanting to have fun in interrupting the sensibility of the crowd. We do not know if this is the case with the quotation just offered. Whether it is or not, the emancipatory discourse raises a question: How far beyond the eloquent babbling of the crowd can such discourse go before it loses any degree of effectiveness? And this question, in turn, raises another one: Is there ever a time when the art of communication should be open to the possibility that a less disruptive, more direct form of communication is best suited for enlightening an audience about contested matters of concern? The art of eloquence serves this purpose. It opts for what Kierkegaard terms a "direct communication" with its audience rather than the practice of "indirect communication" exhibited in the Cubist style of Picasso's paintings, the maieutic artistry at work in the Socratic dialogues, and the disruptive discourse employed by Kierkegaard in defining the self.

Within the early Christian tradition, a classic defense of the art of eloquence is offered by St. Augustine. This art, at its best, serves the truth, which for Augustine ultimately requires that we "leave earthly things and fly back to [God]."[28] Eloquence, however, is not to be forsaken, for it serves a valuable purpose in helping to establish a way for others to come to terms with the Almighty. Augustine puts it this way:

> For since by means of the art of rhetoric both truth and falsehood are urged, who would dare to say that truth should stand in the person of its defenders unarmed against lying, so that they who wish to urge falsehoods may know how to make their listeners benevolent, or attentive, or docile in the presentation, while the defenders of truth are ignorant of that art? Should they speak briefly, clearly, and plausibly while the defenders of truth speak so that they tire their listeners, make themselves difficult to understand and what they have to say? Should they oppose the truth with fallacious arguments and assert falsehoods, while the defenders of truth have

> no ability either to defend the truth or to oppose the false? Should they, urging the minds of their listeners into error, ardently exhort them, moving them by speech so that they terrify, sadden, and exhilarate them, while the defenders of truth are sluggish, cold, and somnolent? Who is so foolish as to think this to be wisdom?[29]

Augustine, of course, is being rhetorical with the instructive questions that he asks here. Christianity needs the art of eloquence to sustain and spread the Word, especially as this homiletic endeavor must take place before so many others whose discourse, although eloquent and entertaining, promotes misunderstandings and falsehoods about the true meaning of the Word. Augustine calls for eloquence to counter this ever-present danger and, in the process, to contribute to an "ecclesiastical literature" that can instruct readers about God's truth and the ways it is best said and practiced.

Kierkegaard takes exception to Augustine's teachings on eloquence, for he finds them contributing to the early decline of authentic Christianity and fostering the crowd-like tendencies of Christendom.[30] The crowd is the untruth. Kierkegaard never tires of making the point: "Something to chatter about! The crowd demands only something to chatter about and this is understood to mean finding something about each other to chatter about, something about our meaningless lives, particularly the trivialities in our lives. Anything else nauseates the public, which knows only one lust—the desire for self-pollution by talking, a lust in which it indulges with the help of the journalist. Journalists are animal-keepers who provide something for the public to talk about. In ancient days people were cast to the wild animals. Now the public devours the people—those tastefully prepared by the journalists."[31]

The chatter of the crowd, its eloquent babbling, deadens our ability to open ourselves to what existence, with its process of becoming and uncertainty, has to teach us about the holiest of matters. Teaching is a calling. Kierkegaard heard the call as a summoning from God requiring the virtue of wholehearted acknowledgment. Acknowledgment is a capacity of consciousness that enables us to remain open to a given matter of concern so that we can admit its wonders into our minds and express to others the understanding we gained and that we believe is worth sharing. Although the intensity of Kierkegaard's acknowledgment of God strained the health of his lived body, it nevertheless was rewarding. He was the individual, the self, that he wanted to be, uncorrupted by others who were content to abide by the ways and means of the crowd. The art of eloquence is not credited with having any value in this situation. Those who have more faith in the educational and civic commitment of this art could turn, for example, to the teachings of Cicero for encouragement: "[W]e are not born for ourselves alone . . . our country claims a share of our being," and if we intend "to contribute to the general good," we must not disparage and retreat from the politics of public life but instead use "our skill, our industry, and our talents to cement human society more closely together man to man." "To be drawn by study away from active life is contrary to moral duty."[32] Although I am confident that Kierkegaard would be overjoyed as individuals, moved by his narrative, joined his cause, I am also confident that he had no desire to be rescued by proponents of the art of eloquence from his way of being true to God. It's the self, not the other, that counts. Kierkegaard created his own world of know-how where anxiety was his constant companion: "the magnitude of anxiety is a prophecy of how wonderful perfection is."[33]

For Kierkegaard, perfection is the self striving to know that which the objective uncertainty of existence makes impossible to know: God. The uncertainty that marks existence calls into question the self's desire for completeness, for perfection. The self is perfectly imperfect.[34] We are back to an oxymoron, a figure of rhetoric, an interruption that is us: the interruption that we are. Anxiety is part of the territory. The emotion makes the self vulnerable to the interruption's defeatist impulse. It also puts the self in touch with the interruption's productive and perfective impulse that inspires the motivation for self-determination and the concerned thought and action that, with the help of a supportive narrative, can better the health of the lived body. Hence Kierkegaard's positive view of "the magnitude of anxiety" and the dignity that it inspires. The health of his lived body is supported by his creation of a narrative that tells how the self's imperfection establishes the perfect way for having faith in God's existence. Although he never puts it this way, the narrative is Kierkegaard's interpretation of what it means to follow God's command "Walk before me and be thou perfect." Existence is structured in such a way as to encourage a belief in God. Kierkegaard supports a theory of intelligent design. His version of this theory justifies living a lonely existence and seeing it as worthwhile and honorable. Indeed, says Kierkegaard, "Ideally speaking it may be perfectly true every man should be given freedom of belief, etc. But what then; where are the men who are spiritually strong enough to be able to use that freedom, who are really capable of standing absolutely alone, alone with God? . . . The man who can really stand alone in the world, only taking counsel from his conscience—that man is a hero."[35] A hero is admired for his or her courage and actions devoted to the well-being of others. I wonder how Kierkegaard saw himself meeting this second requirement.

Kierkegaard stands face to face with the interruption that we are, welcomes the anxiety, and chooses to remain in that situation for as long as he lives. Without his specific interpretation of the dynamics of this interruption, Kierkegaard's version of Christianity would be impossible. Whether this interpretation has any merit is not for me to say. The purpose of my story does not obligate me to do so. Bracketing out the question of God, Kierkegaard does, however, advance an understanding of how the interruption that we are involves a consideration of self-determination, the experience of anxiety, the rhetorical (oxymoronic) nature of the interruption, the crowd-like nature of the world of know-how, and the way in which a certain practice of the art of communication is most truthful to the openness that characterizes our interruptive nature. The art of eloquence and the self's willingness to serve others do not fare especially well in Kierkegaard's religious worldview. The status of this art and its communal function receive more consideration as my story continues with the help of Martin Heidegger. But there is trouble ahead as Heidegger develops his appreciation of these matters.

Martin Heidegger

Heidegger was influenced by the writings of Kierkegaard. He also had a response to the Christian existentialist, which reflected his hesitancy to abide by God-of-the-gaps thinking. "Only from the truth of Being can the essence of the holy be thought. Only from the essence of the holy is the essence of divinity to be thought. Only in the light of the essence of divinity can it be thought or said what the word 'God' is to signify. . . . How can man at the present stage of world history ask at all seriously and rigorously whether the god nears or withdraws, when he has above all neglected to think into the dimension in which alone that question can be asked?"[36]

Heidegger's lifelong project was devoted to answering a specific question: What is the meaning and truth of Being? His book *Being and Time* (1927) changed the course of twentieth-century continental philosophy.

The truth of Being is everywhere to be seen and observed. Being is where the existence of anything shows itself. The truth of Being is an empirical question, and for Heidegger this truth is most apparent in the existence of that being whose consciousness of the world is most advanced in its related capacities of reflection (critical thinking) and articulation (symbolic expression). Heidegger initially puts it this way: Human being "is an entity which does not just occur among other entities. Rather it is optically distinguished by the fact that, in its very Being, that Being is an *issue* for it."[37] In other words, what Heidegger designates as the "special distinctiveness" of human being that differentiates it from other entities is that this entity is concerned with its existence, its Being, its way of becoming what it is. This concern for Being is constantly demonstrated in one's everyday involvements with things and with others. Reflecting on the meaningfulness of what is being demonstrated, one can, and often does (especially in personal crises), raise the question of what it means to be. The question makes explicit a human being's concern for Being. Only a human being is consciously concerned enough to do this. And because it is also capable of understanding to various degrees what it is doing out of concern for its Being, human being can help provide an answer to the question. Heidegger thus tells us that "man should be understood, with the question of Being, as the site which Being requires in order to disclose itself. Man is the site of openness, the there," the place within all of existence where Being finds a "clearing" and whereby it can be seen, observed, and disclosed in language with rigor and care. Demonstrating this receptive response to Being defines for Heidegger "the proper dignity of man."[38]

Heidegger's contribution to advancing our understanding of the interruption that we are emerges as he offers a phenomenological investigation of how a human being provides a clearing for the truth of Being to show itself. His investigation is at times quite similar to what Kierkegaard has to say about the self's authenticity and the way in which the crowd's world of know-how inhibits its appreciation of the essential sermon of existence (the interruption that we are). A brief discussion of Heidegger's take on this latter matter, which is less negative than Kierkegaard's, will be helpful in understanding his assessment of our interruptive nature.

The everyday world of know-how provides a habitat that functions in accordance with societal norms, standards, and well-designed plans that cater to and condition the purposeful and goal directed creatures that we are. Owing to this conditioning, we can become so good at what we are doing that we need not give it a second thought. Take kids to school, pick up Mary and go to work, send emails to customers, grocery shop, call parents, finish painting the guest room. . . . The day is filled with people and places and tools to accomplish tasks. The more smoothly our activities proceed, the more unobtrusively these people, places, and tools present themselves and disappear into their working environments.

As creatures of know-how, we come to see and involve ourselves with the world in an instrumentally oriented manner. The outlook of the world of know-how is that of circumspection, of visualizing and being open to the environment in such a way that it becomes and remains *useful* for our purposes. Here, for example, objects first manifest themselves as equipment, as tools or technologies for accomplishing things.[39] As we wake in the morning and move from the bedroom to the bathroom, beginning the process of going to work, things like the toilet, bath or shower stall, soap, shampoo, razor, and toothbrush present themselves not to the theoretical stare of our speculative eye but rather to the know-how of our well-trained brain and body. A good technology does not call attention to itself. Rather, it withdraws in use and becomes transparent so as not to impede the endeavor that it is helping to facilitate. A shoe that pinches, a pen that skips, a phone connection filled with static, a television without high definition, a computer, Blackberry, or iPad that malfunctions, or a person who shows no respect for proper decorum when communicating with you lack the necessary transparency that would otherwise enhance one's absorption in the performance of some activity. The more inconspicuous the technology or interpersonal interaction, the less we tend to question it. The world of know-how conditions us to leave well enough alone, for here everything and everyone already have their established times, places, and purposes. The everyday world of know-how operates best when matters are going well, remain transparent, uninterrupted, and can thus be easily taken for granted. The more automatic the process, the better it is. Of course, you need to see what you are doing in order to remain preoccupied with your goal-directed activities, but beyond that, there is no good reason for one to fixate on the presence of things, people, and circumstances. The world of know-how favors preoccupation over interruption, habit over disorganization and chaos.

For example, one day your friend John comes to work and looks quite distraught because of family problems at home. His typical ways of being preoccupied with a world of know-how have been interrupted. The next day, however, he is a picture of health. Existential conditions have apparently changed, a world of know-how is back in order, and the change shows itself in the presence of John's lived body. With its brain working, heart beating, and all other physiological mechanisms faring normally, the health of the lived body is as much a matter of personal well-being and public health as it is, for example, a pulse rate of 75 and a blood pressure reading of 120/80. The health of the lived body owes much to a well-ordered and acceptable world of know-how—that communal domain where we develop a self-identity in the midst of and influenced by our being with others.

Heidegger offers us a more positive assessment of the world of know-how than does Kierkegaard. Yet, like Kierkegaard, Heidegger also sees this influential habitat as having a crowd-like tendency to promote a mindless conformism amongst its adherents. Heidegger associates these tendencies with what he terms the "publicness" of "the they." Kierkegaard calls the linguistic practices of the crowd eloquent "babbling." Heidegger calls the linguistic practices of "the they" "idle talk." Commenting on the ways and means of "the they's" world of know-how, Heidegger notes that here "the real dictatorship of the 'they' is unfolded. We take pleasure and enjoy ourselves as they . . . take pleasure; we read, see and judge about literature and art as they see and judge; likewise we shrink back from the 'great mass' as they shrink back, we find 'shocking what they find shocking. . . .' In this averageness with which ["the they"] prescribes what can and may be ventured, it keeps watch over everything exceptional and that thrusts itself to the fore. Every kind of priority gets noiselessly suppressed. Overnight, everything that is primordial gets glossed over as something that has long been well known. Everything gained by a struggle becomes just something to be manipulated."[40] Idle talk fuels the "averageness" of the world of "the they."

Heidegger makes much of how this world, in influencing our self-identity, makes us forgetful of an essential fact of human being: the self's constant "projective" involvement with the temporal process of becoming and understanding its possibilities. This "potentiality-for-Being," a potentiality that constitutes the "not yet" of a person's future development, is what Heidegger terms the "primordial time" of a human being's "authentic temporality," which "lies in advance" of our common everyday understanding of time and is not to be confused with the measured time produced by devices like clocks.[41] The self-identity promoted by our involvement in the world of "the they" is not the authentic self of a human being. Rather, what Heidegger describes as a human being's "own Self" finds its existential origins in this primordial "ability to be," which makes possible one's becoming in the world of "the they" a teacher, husband, Christian, or whatever. For any human being, this ability is uniquely his or her "own." It defines the "authenticity," the most essential truth, of a human being; it forms the temporal basis of the self's historically situated and thus finite freedom, which is always anchored to and constrained by past decisions, present involvements, the self's biological condition, and existing environmental factors.[42]

Heidegger's analysis of the self and temporality echoes what Kierkegaard teaches about these matters. Both see the original functioning of temporality as being more and thus other than a human creation. We did not bring into being the fundamental spatiotemporal structure of existence that "lies in advance" of the calculated time that runs the life of our everyday existence. Kierkegaard credits God as being the creator of this fundamental structure of the self's way of being in the world. Heidegger neither affirms nor denies the claim, for it lies outside his central concern: the question of Being.

Answering the question requires further analysis of the self's authentic temporality. The projective nature of this temporality is constantly calling the self to acknowledge its authenticity and thus to shoulder the responsibility of making thoughtful decisions about how to build and live a meaningful life. The self's authentic temporality features a challenge-response logic. If the self is to remain authentic while living the decisions it made in responding to the challenging call of its fundamental temporality, it must be prepared and willing at any moment to question the supposed correctness of what it is thinking and doing as a result of having made these decisions. The constancy of the challenge-response logic demands as much, for it speaks to the self of uncertainty; the future orientation of existence is forever opening us to the possibility of change, of things being otherwise than usual, of how what is yet to come in our lives may require us, for truth's sake, to rethink and revise what we currently hold to be correct about our circumstances, involvements, and interpretive practices. The constancy of the challenge-response logic is forever calling into question the self's decisive way of being in the world and opening the self to the source of anxiety: the interruption that we are. Abiding by what this call requires, the self is obliged to remain in a continuous state of "struggle" to maintain its authentic way of being-in-the-world.

Human being is its own evocation and provocation. It emits its own challenging call, which demands a heartfelt response. What Heidegger says about the challenge-response logic of the self's authentic temporality is similar to my earlier interpretive assessments of the holy commands "Walk before me and be thou perfect" and "I will give them a heart to know Me that I am the Lord." The self demonstrates perfection when it is true to what its authentic temporality requires it to do. And the self is given a heart—the gift of conscience—so that, at least from a religious perspective, it can know (*scientia*) with (*con*) God. What the self hears and responds to when it displays its perfection for meeting the challenge posed by its authentic temporality is, according to Heidegger, "the call of conscience," which is the result of the dynamic function of the interruption that we are. The call of conscience is this interruption challenging us to make use of its perfective impulse. There is no call of conscience without this perfective impulse.[43] For Heidegger, being exposed to the interruption that we are does not define a moment when the self is positioned to know with God. Rather, the moment marks a time when the self is knowing its own existence, what it is first and foremost before its identity is transformed by the ways and means of the world of know-how dictated by "the they." In Heidegger's terms, the interruption that we are is "the site of openness" that Being requires in order to disclose itself—its meaning and truth. The interruption that we are is the place where the "call of Being" shows itself most clearly. This interruption, which is not a human creation, speaks to us of there being something more than the interruption's challenge-response logic. Human being features an "otherness" that transcends but also informs its existence. For Heidegger, this otherness defines the meaning and truth of Being. Heidegger's ultimate goal is to comprehend as much as possible what this otherness is. He is committed to the task of demonstrating the proper dignity of man. The practice of acknowledgment is the key.

Heidegger's appreciation of this practice adds to our understanding of its function. Acknowledgment is the specific "attunement of consciousness" that most allows for the comprehension of our interruptive nature, as well as the nature of whatever else may direct our attention. "Every affirmation consists in acknowledgment. Acknowledgment lets that toward which it goes come toward it."[44] Acknowledgment is consciousness "releasing" itself from the instrumental and calculative procedures of the world of know-how that typically are at work in our habitual ways of being with things and with others ("the they") and that dictate, for example, how one might unfortunately perceive a severely disabled person as someone whose "life is not worth living." Acknowledgment is consciousness becoming as open-minded as possible to its intended object so to allow for a "'letting be' of what is." Acknowledgment, which Heidegger also considers a "devotional" act associated with the "thanking" capacity of "the heart," widens the cognitive aperture of mere "recognition"; it allows us to be more receptive to someone or something than we are when the matter at hand is known only by a past encounter.[45] Acknowledgment develops the moral potential of recognition. Acknowledgment is that way of "being toward" the world that is most conducive to the process nature of disclosure, whereby something *opens itself* for understanding its truth. The interruption that we are calls for acknowledgment, which focuses our attention on the challenge at hand when interruptions expose us to our interruptive nature. Now we must assume the responsibility of affirming our freedom through resolute choice and thereby become personally involved in the creation of a meaningful existence. Now we must find ways of making use of the perfective impulse of the interruption that we are. Meeting this challenge, whereby the virtue of self-determination (authenticity) is enacted, is how systems of morality (for example, religion) come into being in the first place. The language of morality is the language of responsiveness and responsibility. An earlier stated question comes to mind: Did God create this call of the interruption that we are, or does this call and what it obligates the self to do create God?

Again, Heidegger does not say, but his use of the term "call" is significant. The act of calling is an act of "saying." To say something "means to show and to let [something] be seen." The call of the interruption that we are functions discursively: It has the formal structure of "discourse," which is a mode of disclosure in which something is said, pointed out, revealed, and shared. The call of the interruption that we are is human existence disclosing itself "in silence" to the self living it. This nonverbal act of communication and revelation is what is "talked about" when the interruption calls: the givenness, "the bare 'that it is,'" of the self's existence.[46] Thinking about the interruption that we are in this way allows for the following consideration that affirms a suggestion offered when discussing Kierkegaard's notion of objective uncertainty: The call of the interruption that we are is what ancient Greek rhetorical theory terms epideictic discourse. Such discourse is commonly associated with the employment of language to bestow praise and blame on others. The primary function of epideictic discourse, however, is a "showing forth" (*epideixis*), a disclosing, displaying, saying of the truth of some matter warranting concern. It may thus be said that the interruption that we are is a rhetorical phenomenon. Its discourse calls for decisive and responsible action as the self finds itself in a situation where uncertainty and contingency hold sway. Sounding this call in such a situation is a defining feature of the practice of rhetoric. Indeed, the interruption that we are is a rhetorical phenomenon; its discourse warrants being acknowledged a rhetorical interruption.

Heidegger never speaks of the interruption that we are in this way. He notes, however, that the self's everyday involvement with the world of "the they" must be "interrupted" if the self is to be exposed to and hear the discourse of the interruption that we are.[47] Heidegger offers no discussion of what this interruption can be or why and how it happens. The following example attends to this matter.

A patient seeking a cure for perceived mental problems brings to a psychoanalytic interview a lived experience that has interrupted the patient's everyday existence and that the patient has thought about and made meaningful. In the process, the patient is victimized by what the meaning suggests about the patient's being and the health of his lived body. Specifically, during some moment (or moments) in the patient's lived history, the patient's self, conditioned by his once-stable world of know-how, was understood to be what at the moment was remembered as having-just-been-thus, having-been-thus for a certain period of time, or having-always-been-thus. The patient believes now that what has been will always be. This "what" can be anything disturbing to the patient, anything that suggests to the patient that the remembered behavior is symptomatic of some ailment that will continually be repeated and that the current social mores depict as abnormal. Hence, in seeking the help of the psychoanalyst, the patient is seeking an answer to this question: Is this symptom my truth, what I desire to become (and to be) as a human being?

An interruption has called into question a world of know-how and the health of a lived body that inhabits it. The patient's interpretation of his new state of being forces him to confront another interruption: the interruption that we are and the anxiety that it produces. Here he once again is being interrupted and called into question, making him more susceptible to how members of his once-stable world of know-how will perceive him as ill fitted for their environment. The anxiety is further intensified by how the process of becoming that characterizes his interruptive nature will lead him to continue his dreadful state of being. Heidegger describes this condition as a person not feeling "at home" with his existence, for anxiety opens us to a future where our finitude must come to an end. We are a "Being-towards-death."[48] The business of the psychoanalyst is to listen carefully to the language that the patient uses to describe his plight and to construct a narrative that takes advantage of the productive and perfective impulse of the interruption that we are and that may help the patient find a way that will aid him in thinking differently about his situation and perhaps serve as a remedy for restoring some degree of health to his lived body. The narrative is itself an interruption of an interruption that presently is functioning in a defeatist manner. Heidegger speaks of the "unshakable joy" that can result when the patient is helped to find a way to take advantage of the perfective impulse of the interruption that we are and realize the possibilities he has for bettering his state of existence. Present research in psychiatry confirms that the perfective impulse of the interruption can help a patient use anxiety as a motivational and creative stimulus.[49]

Imagine if Kierkegaard were the patient's psychoanalyst. Anxiety would rule the day as the patient was encouraged to remain being one with the interruption that we are and provided only with a narrative that spoke of the importance of having faith in God. I wonder how comforting that would be for the patient. Selves need a world of know-how as a way of securing degrees of stability in their lives. Yes, a world of know-how can be detrimental to the health of the lived body, but even though it might be perceived as a habitat whose inhabitants are considered abnormal and uncomfortable to be with, it still can serve an invaluable and praiseworthy purpose. I have worked with people who have bipolar disorder and have listened to their family members talk about the effects that the disease has on their lives. The counseling groups and the narratives that are shared define a world of know-how that provides supportive and life-saving care. Worrying about what "the they" will think too often gets in the way. The key is to construct a narrative of self-determination, of authenticity, that facilitates the enactment of the productive and perfective workings of our interruptive nature. It is a way of trying to give people hope rather than leaving them in the clutches of the defeatist impulse of the interruption that we are. It is a virtuous thing to do.

A common criticism of Heidegger's philosophy is that it is too locked into the authenticity of this self-affirming experience, which Heidegger, like Kierkegaard, considers heroic.[50] Heidegger is open to the charge of disparaging the communal nature of human being and the self's responsibility to others. The example just given suggests that matters are not that simple. Heidegger offers a number of insights that indicate that the self's authenticity, which it demonstrates in responding to the call of the interruption that we are, does not lead to an isolationist way of being, as it does in Kierkegaard.

Heidegger is not advocating that his notion of authenticity defines an act that detaches a human being "from its world" such that "it becomes a free-floating 'I.'" On the contrary, the resoluteness associated with the self's authenticity "pushes it into solicitous Being-with-Others." Elaborating on this point, which affirms his understanding that a self's being-in-the-world is always a Being-with-others, Heidegger offers the following important observation: A human being's "resoluteness towards itself is what first makes it possible to let Others who are with it 'be' in their own most potentiality-for-Being, and to codisclose this potentiality in the solicitude which leaps forth and liberates. When [a human being] is resolute, it can become the 'conscience' of Others. Only by authentically Being-their-selves in resoluteness can people authentically be with one another—not by ambiguous and jealous stipulations and talkative fraternizing in the 'they' and in what 'they' want to undertake."[51]

In his later works where he focuses on how "language is the house of Being," Heidegger tells us that "Language has the task of making manifest in its works the existent, and of preserving it as such. In it, what is purest and what is most concealed, and likewise what is complex and ordinary, can be expressed in words. Even the essential word, if is to be understood and so become a possession in common, must make itself ordinary."[52] I know of no rhetorician whose devotion to the art of eloquence and its use of the perfectionist impulse of language to disclose the truth would deny the importance of this claim. It speaks to the relevance of an activity that is essential for demonstrating the proper dignity of human being.

With Heidegger's analysis of the interruption that we are there emerges a consideration of how the resolute self has a responsibility to bring about an authentic community by calling on others to assume the responsibility of affirming their freedom through resolute choice. In doing this, the resolute self not only displays a willingness to test before others the integrity of its affirmed authenticity—a test that the challenge-response logic of the interruption that we are requires us to take time and again—but also engages others in the related tasks of trying to cultivate all that is good in their "heritage," so that they too might have a say in establishing their collective "destiny." Summarizing this entire process, Heidegger notes: "Only in communicating and in struggling [with others] does the power of destiny become free."[53]

The struggle here requires the self to open itself to others by becoming thoughtful and respectful of their rights, circumstances, and feelings, allowing them time to share their interpretation of the issues at hand, and joining them in trying to find the most fitting and telling words for communicating what is believed to be the truth in question. In short, the self owes the other what Heidegger terms "considerateness." The self must demonstrate this virtue if it is "to let Others who are with it 'be' in their ownmost potentiality-for-Being." And this, in turn, might require the virtue of great patience—what Heidegger terms "forbearance"—on the part of the self, since what others have to say in response may indicate that they do not understand or misunderstand what they are being told or that they perhaps find the self guilty of maintaining a wrong point of view.[54] Trying to build an authentic community can be a time-consuming task filled with controversy. When such controversy arises, the practice of public moral argument is called for as a fair-minded course of action.

Nevertheless, according to Heidegger, it is essential that the self listen carefully to the other, for the virtue of "listening to . . . is [the self's] existential way of Being-open as Being-with for Others."[55] Being open and listening to others is how the self counters the selfish tendency of becoming so engrossed in figuring out what it wants to express next that it misses or forgets what others are expressing. Authentic community is built not on egoism but on the altruism of being "for Others" and on the "empathy" that this makes possible. Heroism on the part of the authentic self precludes selfishness, which inhibits the self collaborating with others whereby the perfectionist use of language might develop as the involved parties struggle to disclose the truth of some matter of concern.

Creating and maintaining authentic community is a virtuous activity—the ultimate goal of the tradition of civic republicanism. Robert Bellah and his colleagues summarize the teachings of this tradition: "[C]ommunity means a solidarity based on a responsibility to care for others because that is essential to living a good life." Moreover, civic republicanism, emphasizing as it does the importance of developing a rhetorically competent citizenry, maintains that the authenticity of "public life is built upon the . . . languages and practices of commitment that shape character. These language and practices establish a web of interconnection by creating trust, joining people to families, friends, communities, and churches, and making each individual aware of his reliance on the larger society. They form those habits of the heart that are the matrix of a moral ecology, the connecting tissue of a body politic."[56] The interruption that we are is not just about the self. It also calls the self to attend to the other, especially when the self, in maintaining its authenticity, seeks input and critique from those who are involved in a discursive transaction with the self and who know that the self will listen and welcome whatever controversy may materialize. The philosopher Henry W. Johnstone speaks of the commitment that is required here:

> The individual who attempts to speak and act in such a way as to remain true to himself must come into radical conflict with others no less true to themselves but according to different beliefs. He cannot sidestep the conflict merely by withdrawing the expression of his beliefs. Such sudden silence might attend the comic downfall of a buffoon, but could not be the choice of a person of integrity. Nor can such an individual overcome the conflict by using violence to annihilate the opposition. Action of that sort would bring down a tragic fate, for one does not express one's commitment at all except in communicating it to others capable of taking issue with it. The idea of expression without an interlocutor is just as incoherent as that of commitment without expression.[57]

In speaking of the need to "come into radical conflict with others," Johnstone identifies interruption as a necessary event for testing a person's true character and wisdom. *How* this interruption is communicated and expressed defines the event as having a rhetorical nature. As Johnstone notes, "*Rhetoric is the evocation and the maintenance of the consciousness required for communication.*"[58] The interruption that we are calls for the art of eloquence.

Heidegger is not unaware of the importance of how rhetoric can help achieve the goal of creating and maintaining authentic community. In 1924 he devoted an entire semester seminar to Aristotle's *Rhetoric,* finding in this text key directives for understanding how a concern for Being shows itself in our everyday communal existence.[59] The noted classical and rhetorical scholar Nancy S. Struever maintains that, as seen in his lecture manuscript, Heidegger's interpretation of the *Rhetoric* "remains, arguably, the best twentieth century reading" of the text.[60] Heidegger knows the importance of developing our rhetorical competence such that we might maintain and improve the sociopolitical workings and well-being of our communal existence. The genuine function of such competence extends beyond mere persuasion to include the development of judgment (*krisis*) and practical wisdom (*phronesis*). Rhetorical competence lends itself to collaborative deliberation and reflective inquiry (including the self-deliberation of the individual). In the rhetorical situation an audience is not set at a distance. Rather, it is acknowledged, engaged, and called into the space of practical concerns as the orator works to establish an emotional connection with the audience and its immediate concerns and interests. Knowing how to stir the soul rhetorically is essential because existential questions concerning the livelihood of a community are not usually decided with the equations of demonstrations or the syllogisms of dialectic. Existence is a gamble based on probabilities, and the emotional outlook of the hoi polloi influences their judgment at the time the bet is placed. If rhetoric is to perform its most worthy function of trying to move people toward the good and the truth, it must cast a concerned and knowing eye on the emotional character of those whom it wishes to move. A moving of the passions is a sine qua non of persuasion; truth alone is not sufficient to guide the thoughtful actions of human beings.

I am making much of where Heidegger's notions of "communicating" and "struggling" can lead us in appreciating the nature, scope, and function of the interruption that we are. Heidegger offers a more supportive and advanced understanding of how the interruption that we are, the self's authenticity, rhetoric, and the creation of authentic community can work hand in hand than does Kierkegaard. Still, things can go terribly wrong when the call of the interruption that we are is heard and the self's response distorts Heidegger's directives. Heidegger is a tragic case in point.

Volume 1 of Adolf Hitler's anti-Semitic *Mein Kampf* was published in 1925. Volume 2 was published in 1926. On January 30, 1933, German president Paul von Hindenburg appointed Hitler chancellor of Germany. The Holocaust was now officially under way. On February 1 Hitler gave his "Proclamation to the German People" in Berlin. On March 15 he proclaimed the Third Reich. On March 20 Dachau, the first Nazi concentration camp, was completed, opening March 22. On March 23 the Reichstag passed the Enabling Act, making Hitler dictator of Germany. On April 1 the Nazis mandated a boycott of Jewish shops and businesses. On April 26 the Gestapo was established in Germany. On May

10 the Nazis staged massive public book burnings throughout Germany. On May 26 the Nazi Party introduced a law to legalize eugenic sterilization. On May 27 Heidegger gave his address as the newly elected rector of Freiburg University.[61] He had already joined the National Socialist Party, believing that his investigations into the meaning of Being could become the "true" guiding vision for the party's political mission of restoring Germany's "spiritual" status, which had been in steep economic, political, and social decline since the horrors of World War I. For Heidegger, issues like eugenic sterilization missed the point. The question of Being was not a biological and racial issue. The rhetorical situation in which Heidegger found himself forced him to discover a way to accommodate his philosophy with a political practice that, at the time and thereafter, showed no inclination for following the type of thinking that Heidegger commended in his extant and future writings. The rhetorical situation exposed Heidegger to the interruption that we are and the need to make use of the interruption's perfective impulse. The health of a lived body was at stake. A troublesome narrative was forthcoming.

A major theme of the address is the importance of maintaining one's authenticity by personally assuming the burden of freedom that comes with making some resolute choice about matters of importance. Another major theme is the urgency of acknowledgment. If *das Volk* are to make resolute decisions that are well informed, wise, and responsible, they must be as open as possible to and acknowledge the truth of what demands attention now.

Heidegger emphasizes that acknowledgment is "the essence of science" and that "all science is philosophy, whether it knows and wills it—or not" (6–7). The claim reflects Heidegger's phenomenological proclivities: Philosophy is valued for its empirical capacity to direct us toward "the things themselves" such that we can "let them be" what they are, thereby allowing them to "speak" their being, their truth. Philosophical inquiry is thereby legitimized by equating it with an academic endeavor well known and respected for its dedication to knowledge and progress: things that are much needed by the German people in 1933. Fulfilling this need calls for what Heidegger describes as "the strength for leadership": "For what is decisive in leading is not just walking ahead of others but the strength to be able to walk alone, not from obstinacy or a craving for power, but empowered by the deepest purpose and the broadest obligation. Such strength binds to what is essential, selects the best, and awakens the genuine following of those who have new courage" (9).

Heidegger finds this leadership at work with the "German students [who] are on the march . . . seeking . . . those leaders [for example, Hitler, Heidegger] through whom they want to elevate their own purpose so that it becomes a grounded, knowing truth, and to place it into the clarity of interpretive and effective word and work" (9–10). Under the guidance of dedicated teachers, the students thus supply what Heidegger terms "Labor Service" to the state. Such service takes on a much needed "Military" dimension: "It demands the readiness, secured by knowledge and skill and tightened by discipline, to give the utmost in action" (10). Hence, by way of Labor and Military Service, the students act to provide "Knowledge Service" to the state, which is now in the best position to define its own destiny. These services serve to bridge the genuine mission of the university to the political realm and, supposedly, to ensure that this realm is true to its destiny for possible greatness. To ensure that these services are continuously working together, Heidegger insists that students and teachers must be willing to "confront one another, ready for *battle*": "All abilities of will and thought, all strengths of the heart, and all capabilities of the body must be *through* battle, heightened *in* battle, and preserved *as* battle" (12). Heidegger aligns this process with the "essential opposition" between "leading and following" that must take place in the educational environment (12–13). Importantly, for Heidegger, students and teachers must jointly assume the responsibility of being both leaders and followers. "Battle alone keeps this opposition open and implants in the entire body of teachers and students that basic attitude" of acknowledgment that must be at work in a people's "struggle" for authenticity (13). Battle occurs when the related services of labor, the military, and knowledge acquisition are hard at work.

Heidegger's rectorial address is filled with the rhetoric of National Socialism: Labor and Military service; battle and struggle [*Kampf*], also translated as "conflict"; new courage; students on the march; leaders and followers. The rhetoric is somewhat tempered by an allegiance to the rightful role of the university in cultivating acknowledgment, science, and truth. Criticized for how this rhetorical tactic left too much room for interpreting his words as favoring the political options of Hitler's brand of National Socialism, Heidegger would later argue in his *An Introduction to Metaphysics* that the "works being peddled about nowadays as the philosophy of National Socialism" have nothing whatever to do with what Heidegger considered, contra Hitler, to be the "the inner truth and greatness of this movement": what it has to teach us about the "encounter between global technology and modern man" and how this encounter is lessening our capacity to hear the call of Being.[62] Heidegger argues further that whenever he refers to such politically loaded terms as "battle," "conflict," and "struggle," he is echoing what the ancient Greek philosopher Heraclitus (535 B.C.E.) posited with his theory of "conflict or opposition," which he associates with the presence of the Logos—the way reality presents and discloses itself and thereby "speaks" of what and how it is.[63] Heidegger was a philosopher dedicated to advancing the fundamental teachings of some of his ancient philosophical ancestors, not a politician favoring Hitler's Aryan dream. Still, Heidegger remained a National Socialist after the war, though he never retreated from the position that this movement was vacuous and dangerous without the guidance of philosophers who, like himself, were dedicated to hearing the call, knowing the truth of Being, and rectifying the movement that had come to power in 1933.

We learn something of the Nazi reaction to Heidegger's teachings by listening to the complaints of Nazi ideologues like Erick Jaensch, who in 1934 maintained that Heidegger's philosophy, with its hairsplitting distinctions, is similar to Talmudic thought, holds "extraordinary fascination" for Jews, and is the product of a disintegrative mind "on the border-line between mental health and illness."[64] The Nazis perceived Heidegger as rhetorically, politically, morally, and psychologically incompetent. His perspective of his country's destiny was far too philosophical and misdirected for the political exigencies at hand. The same criticism, however, comes from the political left, which, for example, read Heidegger's ambiguous use of words as selling out to a crazed eugenic movement. Moreover, the criticism also encourages us to wonder why Heidegger's authentic desire for disclosing the truth failed to acknowledge in more specific and concrete terms what he undoubtedly knew about Hitler's controversial orders months before Heidegger gave his address. There was, indeed, the "Jewish Question" (*Die Judenfrage*), which was very much a part of the historical, moral, and rhetorical situation present at the time.[65]

To speak favorably of this question would have been courageous but also quite destructive for Heidegger's personal and professional life. Was Heidegger a coward? An incredible egotist? A survivor? He certainly was a nationalist, and scholars agree that he was fanatical when it came to his devotion to philosophy. Unlike many of his colleagues, he chose not to leave the Fatherland. In so doing, he demonstrated a lack of morally wise political judgment. Moreover, his attempt to be rhetorically competent proved disastrous.

The philosophical and political ambiguity of Heidegger's rhetoric opens the door for accusations that, at the very least, he is guilty by association with the Nazi program of eugenics. Heidegger did not support this horribly nihilistic program, but neither did he explicitly acknowledge its evil. Instead, he merely equated it in 1949 with a specific effect of technological progress: "Agriculture is now a motorized food industry, the same thing in its essence as the production of corpses in the gas chambers and the extermination camps, the same thing as blockades and the reduction of countries to famine, the same thing as the manufacture of atomic bombs."[66]

The moral and rhetorical inappropriateness of this claim is obvious. Heidegger's perfectionist use of language is a sham. For the particular showing forth of death in question calls for witnesses who can use rhetoric that becomes itself a showing forth of what is—an epideictic event that is moving (rightly emotional) enough to have its witnesses realize how dreadful the consequences can be when people know not how to take to heart the presence and cries of others who would have us never forget what was done to them. Recall that in the Bible one reads: "I will give them a heart to know Me, that I am the Lord" (Jeremiah 24:7). The gift here is that of conscience: the capacity to remain open to (acknowledge) and be awed and instructed by the happenings and mysteries of life. Heidegger had time to see what was happening to those who did not fit the Aryan vision of the *Ubermensch*; he had time to leave Germany; he had time to acknowledge what he eventually described simply as his "own inadequacy" as a philosopher blinded for the moment by a ruinous political ideology.[67] Where was Heidegger's conscience, his heartfelt concern, as he spoke about the call of Being and the self-assertion of the German university at a time when a competently created work of epideictic rhetoric was desperately needed to instruct the thinking and actions of others who lived on during and after the Holocaust? Heidegger's rhetoric was far too limited in reaching out to and acknowledging other German citizens whose marginalization would become catastrophic.

This limitation is especially important when considering a thinker such as Heidegger. He maintains that the essential character of language lies in its "saying" power, its capacity to disclose matters of concern by showing us their unique meaning and significance. This disclosing function of language allows us to associate it with the power to show and speak to some extent the truth of whatever is being talked about. Truth is first and foremost a process of disclosure. We define things to understand what they are (in truth). Communication and struggling with others is a way of facilitating this process, which, as Heidegger emphasizes in *Being and Time,* allows for the creation of authentic community. The authentic self is obligated to engage in this rhetorical process so to test the truthfulness of whatever it claims to be right and just. Moreover, the authentic self is obligated to demonstrate considerateness and forbearance when listening to responses to its stated position. Heidegger failed to hear and respond in an authentic way to the call of the interruption that we are and the demands it makes regarding the ethical practice of rhetoric. Heidegger's character was void of the proper dignity of man.

The range of his phenomenological commitment to "letting beings be," to letting them "speak for themselves," and to acknowledging all that they have to say lacked scope and generosity. The beings in question were the Jews and other non-Aryan and "unfit" populations. Heidegger never acknowledges their "voice" in his writings, and this voice had its own truths to tell. Heidegger failed the test of listening to others. Managed by a Nazi rhetoric housed in a world of know-how that qualified as being but a habitat for a monstrous "they," these truths remained concealed and distorted. Sadly, with the 2014 translation of his "Black Book Diaries," which he began writing in 1931, there is clear evidence that Heidegger included the "Jews" in those populations that were destroying the traditional cultural and rural heritage of Germany that Heidegger cherished.[68]

Given his description of "the they," Heidegger could have said something like this: "Culturally, he contaminates art, literature, the theater, makes a mockery of natural feeling, overthrows all concepts of beauty and sublimity, of the noble and the good, and instead drags men down into the sphere of his own base nature." These are the words of Adolph Hitler, contained in his *Mein Kampf*.[69] What Heidegger discloses in *Being and Time* about the interruption that we are reveals numerous insights and directives that can be used for cultivating the good of humankind. In 1933, however, Heidegger distorted these insights and directives. He allowed the idle talk of a fascist "they" to confuse his understanding of who "the they" truly is. The Nazi world of know-how fits the bill. Who exactly is Heidegger referring to in *Being and Time* when he speaks of the other, who the self is obligated to acknowledge as an interlocutor and potential critic of the self's authenticity? Heidegger doesn't say, beyond referring to this human being in an extremely abstract way. The Jewish people are an other. They certainly qualify as such, based on Heidegger's discussion of what communication and struggle, forbearance and consideration entail. If one takes exception to the other's way of being, does that disqualify the other as a person who warrants the affirming acknowledgment that Heidegger recommends in *Being and Time?* Heidegger never admits as much in the pages of this book.

The phenomenologist and Talmudic scholar Emmanuel Levinas, a student and unrelenting critic of Heidegger, credits *Being and Time* as being a "great event of our century."[70] Levinas also tells us that Heidegger's incredibly sparse remarks concerning the other, and especially his forgetfulness of the topic in his political engagements, are unforgettable and unforgiveable. I agree. Like many others, however, I remain convinced that in the thinking of this philosopher there is much that is valuable for conducting a phenomenological analysis of the Being of human existence and, for my particular purpose, understanding the nature, scope, and function of the interruption that we are.[71] Heidegger moves us beyond Kierkegaard's understanding of our interruptive nature by offering a more extensive assessment of a human being's relationship with truth, human dignity, acknowledgment, the world of know-how, and how the self's authenticity, aided by the practice of rhetoric, has a crucial role to play in cultivating the health of the lived body and fostering the communal existence of our being-with-and-for-others. The relationship with others requires the self to listen to what they have to say and to demonstrate considerateness and forbearance in their presence. The self is obligated to have others question its position on contested issues. *Being and Time* commends virtues that inform the noble character of human being. The importance of these virtues is strikingly clear when they are absent in situations where they are desperately needed.

If only Heidegger had remained true in 1933 to what *Being and Time* allows us to understand about the interruption that we are and what it calls us to do.

If only Heidegger had offered a more morally robust appreciation of the other. Indeed, if only Heidegger had accomplished these tasks, then the author of *Being and Time,* this great event in twentieth-century philosophy, could have avoided an ever-growing amount of criticism undermining this author's character and career. Levinas is famous for advancing this criticism by way of his highly influential ethical philosophy of the other. The philosophy advances our understanding of the moral nature of the interruption that we are, although deficiencies exist in his treatment of the topic. Ironically, these deficiencies are associated with what we learn from Kierkegaard and Heidegger about the self's authenticity.

CHAPTER 3

Existence and the Other

"To be for the Other is to be good."

Emmanuel Levinas, *Totality and Infinity*

Consider this scenario: Your significant other's birthday is tomorrow. You inhabit a world of know-how whose rules, routines, and habits dictate that the proper thing to do is to purchase a card that indicates that you remembered this once-a-year event. It is a nice thing to do. Acknowledgment! You go to the store, survey the card rack until you find a card or two that contain words that you find fitting. You purchase the cards. Expectations have been met. You have done your job. You're happy. Your significant other will be happy. A self is serving the other. The health of your lived body is in good shape. The narrative of a world of know-how lives on.

There are, however, other worlds of know-how informed by narratives that would find your efforts to be a waste of time and money and exceptionally short-sighted. If you really loved your significant other, you would compose a handwritten letter that demonstrates your skill in the art of eloquence. Such a letter is far more thoughtful and personal than the manufactured words that are copied on thousands of pieces of cardboard by a machine. Certainly a loved one deserves more than such a mechanical product. It's the difference between recognition and acknowledgment. Or, better yet, forget the letter and enhance the acknowledgment. Sit down with your loved one and spend the time sharing your wholehearted feelings about how much she or he means to you. Put yourself on the line. The art of eloquence is demanding. Sure, the communicating and struggle might be difficult as you stumble trying to find the right words, the perfect words. Tears might flow. Considerateness and forbearance would have no limits. "I couldn't live without you!" Can a self serve the other more than that? A teaching of Judaism is on your side: "The deepest wisdom man can attain is to know that his destiny is to aid, to serve [the other]. . . . The aspiration is to obtain; the perfection is to dispense."[1]

Of course, your significant other might bring to the scene another ruled world of know-how and complicate the situation: "Hey, this is all I get for my birthday? Where's the cake? Where's the present? Are we going out to dinner? And where's the card?" Your world of know-how has suffered a significant interruption. The health of your lived body is in question. You are headed in the direction of coming face to face with the interruption that we are. But at least your intentions were noble, virtuous, and dignified. You are a self that sought to serve the other. And you are an other who was mistreated by a self. Although it might not serve as much consolation, Levinas would shake your hand. The self's devotion to the other is unbounded. Levinas's philosophy develops a narrative devoted to affirming this point. The narrative encourages us to revise somewhat our present understanding of the nature, scope, and function of the interruption that we are. Before I do this, however, I want to discuss how Levinas conceives what our card-giver has to face as he or she confronts this interruption.

Levinas

According to Levinas, "Everyday existence is a preoccupation with salvation."[2] What we seek salvation from is the very thing that Heidegger associated with the ultimate source of anxiety—the interruption that we are—but that he also claimed can elicit unshakable joy on our part. Levinas admits that it is the self, not the other, that confronts the interruption that we are. "I am not the other. I am all alone. It is the being in me, the fact that I exist, my existing, that constitutes the absolutely intransitive element, something without intentionality or relationship. One can exchange everything between beings except existing."[3] In this sense, to be by nature a creature whose everyday life is always caught up in relationships with things and with others still leaves something that only the self can call its own and that is the source of what Heidegger defines as a human being's "authenticity." The self exists, and in and through this existing it is the self that, in a moment of great anxiety or immense joy, must constantly take on the personal challenge of the interruption that we are by affirming its freedom through resolute choice.

When Levinas speaks of the interruption that we are, he more often than not emphasizes its "darker" side, its destructive and defeatist function. This interruption "is essentially alien and strikes against us. We undergo its suffocating embrace like the night, but it does not respond to us. There is pain in Being."[4] We experience this pain whenever we are forced to come face to face with the interruption that we are, or what Levinas terms "the indissoluble unity between the existent and existing."[5] This unity, according to Levinas, defines the most primordial form of solitude or aloneness that can be experienced by human beings. "Solitude is the very unity of the existent, the fact that there is something in existing starting from which existence occurs. The subject is alone because it is one with its Being [the interruption that we are] . . . it cannot detach itself from itself" and remain alive to be what it is.[6] Levinas describes this state of being as one of "suffering." In this state of being, "there is an absence of all refuge. It is the fact of being directly exposed to being. It is made up of the impossibility of fleeing or retreating. The whole acuity of suffering lies in this impossibility of retreat. It is the fact of being backed up against life and being": the interruption that we are.[7]

I see little difference between what Levinas is suggesting here and what Heidegger has to say about anxiety and the defeatist impulse of the interruption that we are. The example of the patient in psychoanalysis, presented in chapter 2, speaks to the issue. Levinas admits, however, that there is a lighter side to our interruptive nature.

For Heidegger, the awesomeness of coming face to face with this interruption is associated not only with its being a source of anxiety for the self but also with how it functions to encourage the self to take control of its life. The interruption has a dark side, but it also is structured so to allow us to be joyful about what we can do to improve our existence. The interruption that we are exhibits a productive and perfective impulse: Its challenge-response logic calls the self to better itself whenever an interruption exposes the self to its interruptive nature. Levinas agrees. Although he maintains that the solitude of the self brings it pain, he admits that "a solitude is necessary in order for there to be a freedom of beginning, the existent's mastery over existing—that is, in brief, in order for there to be an existent. Solitude is not only a despair and an abandonment, but also a virility, a pride and sovereignty."[8] For Levinas, this capacity should be understood as indicating that along with the pain, solitude, and suffering that is caused by the interruption that we are, there comes "the love of life"—a love that is, in fact, presupposed by the darker side of the interruption. Here is how Levinas puts it: "At the origin there is a being gratified, a citizen of paradise. The 'emptiness' felt implies that the need which becomes aware of it abides already in the midst of an enjoyment—be it that of the air one breathes. It anticipates the joy of satisfaction, which is better than ataraxy. Far from putting the sensible life into question, pain takes place within its horizon and refers to the joy of living. Already and henceforth life is loved."[9] The love of life is the productive and perfective impulse of the interruption that we are. The issue here is the self, not the other. Neither the self or the other would exist without the interruption that we are.

But all of this is too Heideggerian for Levinas. He is not interested in the dynamics of the interruption that we are. Rather, he finds another interruption to have greater importance for the self and its relationship to the other. Later I suggest how his slighting of the self's relationship with its interruptive nature raises problems for Levinas's philosophy of the other. What this philosophy teaches us about interruption is, however, invaluable for my story.

We exist in a world of otherness (alterity), of all that is but that is not ourselves. Otherness is a fact of life. Levinas is interested primarily in how this otherness shows itself in the face of the other and how it instructs who we are as ethical beings. As a phenomenologist, Levinas begins his investigations where he must—in the everyday social world where the presence of others (even when they are absent) is a given, a fact of life. Levinas terms this givenness "proximity," that primordial temporal and spatial relationship between the self and the other that is always there before one even knows, for example, that for the past two minutes the person standing three feet to your left has been taken with your presence. Levinas's specific term for the presence of the other (and the self, which is also an other to other selves) is the "face," or what he defines as "the expressive in the Other (and the whole human body is in this sense more or less face)."[10] Elsewhere he writes, "A face has a meaning not by virtue of the relationship in which it is found, but out of itself; that is what expression is. A face is the presentation of an entity as an entity, its personal presentation . . . the existence of a substance, a thing in itself."[11] What Levinas offers here is a strict phenomenological analysis. When he refers to the face as "expression," he is simply substituting a word that in Heideggerian phenomenology is described as the "presencing," "disclosing," "saying," or "showing-forth" of some object of concern. The face, in other words, defines an epideictic event. Much is made of this event in Jewish thought, which is an essential element of Levinas's philosophy. Consider, for example, the words of Rabbi Abraham Heschel: "A human being has not only a body but also a face. A face cannot be grated or interchanged. A face is a message, a face speaks, often unbeknown to a person. Is not the human face a living mixture of mystery and meaning? We are all able to see it, and are all unable to describe it. . . . The most exposed part of the body, it is the least describable, a synonym for an incarnation of uniqueness. Can we look at a face as if it were a commonplace?"[12]

Levinas offers a condensed description of the face when he tells us that "the face speaks." This discursive act operates as an instance of the dynamic function of showing. Hence, the face speaks a primordial discourse whose reality is not a human creation. Rather, this disclosing of the face is the basis of the everyday discourse of language that we employ to structure and make meaningful our social and political existence. It is this discourse—Levinas terms it the "said"—that allows us to describe how the face speaks—Levinas terms it the "saying." Levinas would thus have us understand that the "Face and discourse are tied. The face speaks. It speaks, it is in this that it renders possible and begins all discourse."[13] What Levinas says about this primordial discursive act is no different from what Heidegger says about the original saying and showing of the interruption that we are.

The primordial discourse that the face speaks defines what Levinas describes as the original "event of communication" that occurs between the other and the self. The event is nonverbal communication in its most original form, unless you consider the nonverbal communication that comes from the interruption that we are. The difference, however, is important. Levinas is talking about the self-other relationship, not the self's relationship with its own interruptive nature. The face speaks, and the self is made aware of an "exposure" (a showing) of otherness coming from the presence of the other. Levinas refers to this evocative event as "the epiphany of the face" from which emerges a "call of conscience." The importance of this call and its educational value cannot be overemphasized in Levinas's philosophy. The call defines an act of "teaching" that informs the self about the status of its existence and its obligation to serve the other. Levinas offers what I take to be his most explicit description of this process when he notes: "I am defined as a subjectivity, a particular person, as an 'I' [or self], precisely because I am exposed to the other. It is my inescapable and incontrovertible answerability to the other that makes me an individual 'I.' So that I become a responsible or ethical 'I' to the extent that I agree to depose or dethrone myself—to abdicate my position of centrality—in favor of the vulnerable other. . . . The ethical 'I' is subjectivity precisely in so far as it kneels before the other, sacrificing its own liberty *to the more primordial call of the other*. . . . I can never escape the fact that the other has demanded a response from me before I affirm my freedom not to respond to his demand."[14]

The call of conscience is interruptive: It calls into question the self's egotistic tendencies and know-it-all attitudes that preoccupy the self with its own well-being rather than with the immediate and perhaps long-term life-affirming needs of the other. The face speaks this interruption with its discourse. Levinas characterizes this primordial discourse as a "rhetoric without eloquence."[15] The description is fitting, given that Levinas is talking about a discourse that, without the presence of the art of eloquence, displays a rhetorical impulse to address a self that is expected to respond to the call of the other.[16] For Levinas, unlike Heidegger, conscience (con-scientia) is a self knowing-with the other, not a self knowing-with itself.

The call of conscience instigates a "moving out of oneself" toward the Other.[17] Being-with others would be nothing more than an adventure in power, violence, and survival of the fittest if it were not for the fact that, at its most primordial level, human existence is not only a temporal happening (a Being-unto-death) but something whose unfolding is directed toward the other. Having failed to appreciate the intricacies of this movement, Heidegger, according to Levinas, did not see how its direction of "one to another," of "one for another," defines a fundamental existential event, a "being-for others," out of which any particular act of moral acknowledgment is born. The indelible communal character of human existence is made possible by an altruistic and thus moral impulse that lies at the heart of human being. This point is crucial for understanding the nature, scope, and function of the interruption that we are: *The interruptive nature of our existence entails a moral function. In the process of becoming what is not yet in its existence, the self is always on the way toward the other.* This finding is a significant contribution to the story of how interruption is an essential feature of human existence. Heidegger completely misses the point. Notice, however, that the contribution makes no sense without acknowledging the equally essential feature of the interruption that we are.

Levinas emphasizes that the movement of the self toward the other is "asymmetrical" and defines the "primordial domain of ethics." He makes much of how reciprocity is not a requirement in this domain. The self finds its existence, its subjectivity, to be defined first and foremost by its inevitable ethical obligation to respond to the other's demand for acknowledgment. The call of conscience requires nothing less than this altruistic and respectful way of being, which for Levinas is the defining feature of human dignity. Levinas employs biblical discourse supposedly first uttered by God and responded to by Adam to emphasize further the importance of the demand: "Where art thou?" "Here I am!"[18] The call of conscience and what it requires brings to mind another relevant and fitting segment of Scripture: "Walk before me and be thou perfect." Responding to the call's demand to fulfill its obligation to serve the other, the self assumes the task of perfecting itself, which for Levinas warrants acclaim for its goodness. Goodness is the ongoing call of conscience that lies at the heart of human existence and that forever calls the self into question. "Goodness in the subject is anarchy itself," a constant interruption that raises this moral issue: Are you being just in all that you say and do?[19] The face speaks. "Where art thou? Goodness makes it possible to say 'Here I am!'" Goodness brings the self and other closer together. Goodness promotes neighborhood: "The Other becomes my neighbor precisely through the way the face summons me, calls for me, begs for me, and in so doing recalls my responsibility, and calls me into question."[20] A demonstration of human dignity is expected.

Answering an earlier asked question furthers an appreciation of our goodness: What would your life be like if no one acknowledged your existence? The question confronts one with the possibility of social death: being isolated, marginalized, ignored, and forgotten by others. The unacknowledged find themselves in an "out-of-the-way" place where it is hard for human beings, given their social instinct, to feel at home. Levinas has this fate in mind when, turning once again to biblical inspiration, he discusses how the face speaks a specific all important commandment: "Thou shall not commit murder."[21] The commandment is justified by how the self is obligated to be open to and acknowledge the other.

The discourse of the commandment (a saying) makes sense as Levinas converts it to his discourse (a said). That is the best that one can do: employing the perfectionist impulse of language to make the said as true to the saying as possible. Hence, following Levinas throughout his works, we understand that the commandment does not only mean that the self should not kill others. Rather, the term "murder" also refers to an action that negates the self's potential to respect and meet the needs of others whose circumstances put them in harm's way. The biblical story of Moses and the Exodus of the Jewish people from ancient Egypt, for example, illustrates how one can avoid murdering the other. The story warns against the injustice of allowing for social death and worse. Goodness remedies this injustice and the suffering it engenders.

Drawing from his Jewish heritage, Levinas appropriates biblical material to articulate a said that he believes is more instructive, more elucidating, for coming to terms with the saying of the face and its otherness. Levinas maintains that "we Westerners, from California to the Urals, [are] nourished by the Bible as much as by the Presocratics" and the ancient tradition of Greek philosophy.[22] The face speaks. What it has to say, what it commands, has Levinas claim that "the other must be closer to God than I."[23] The other warrants this status given what it shows itself to be. The showing of the face of the other offers a particular display of the otherness that is an essential feature of reality. Otherness is itself something more than a human creation. Otherness is transcendent. The otherness of God is the ultimate occurrence of transcendence. The otherness displayed in the face of the other exposes and expresses a "trace" of how it is that God presents Itself to humankind. Standing face to face with the other, we are privy to a saying that grants the possibility that God, the "Wholly Other," may "come to mind" as transcendence, which Levinas associates with "[God's] semantics." With what the face has to show and say, we can hear something of God's "infinite" presence and "Word"; we can think "a thought which thinks more than it thinks, beyond what it thinks."[24]

Levinas's discussion of God is consistent with the priority he grants to the other over the self, which exists to serve the other. As noted, Levinas maintains that the relationship is asymmetrical. Beyond responding "Here I am" to the other's call of "Where art thou?," reciprocity has no role to play in the relationship. The self is there to serve the other, not the other way around. This being the case, Levinas's claim that his overall project constitutes a "philosophy of dialogue" is rather odd.[25] Dialogue is an activity of reciprocity. Levinas addresses the problem in his later philosophy when he admits that "'Thanks to God', I am another for the others."[26] The self deserves from the other what the other deserves from the self. With dialogue as our goal, we exist not merely as a self or an other but rather as a self/other. Levinas does not employ this construction, although I believe it is appropriate for describing what Levinas terms "the third":

those individuals who have something to advocate in situations where the truth of matters of interest are being contested and thus where arguments are bound to happen between self/others who demand reciprocity from their interlocutors. For Levinas, such situations allow for the promotion of "justice," which makes possible the creation of civil society and laws that, at least for the time being, grant guidelines for the righteousness of interpersonal behavior. Levinas puts it this way: "There is a certain measure of violence necessary in terms of justice, but if one speaks of justice, it is necessary to allow judges, it is necessary to allow institutions and the state . . . to live in a world of citizens [self/others], and not only in the order of the Face to Face."[27]

This is not to say, however, that the ethical directives reflected in the dynamics of the Face to Face should be denied equal status in organizing and regulating the social and political affairs of the world of citizens. What needs to be determined in this case is the applicability of theory to practice. In a rare practical example that illustrates the applicability of his philosophy, Levinas notes: "I remember meeting once with a group of Latin American students of Marxist liberation and terribly concerned by the suffering and unhappiness of their people in Argentina." During the dialogical exchange, the students asked him "rather impatiently if [he] had ever actually witnessed the utopian rapport with the other which [his] ethical philosophy speaks of." He replied: "Yes, indeed, here in this room."[28]

With what I have discussed so far about Levinas's philosophy, I think it is fair to say that the students heard a call of conscience coming from others. They are acknowledging this call and what it demands: Accept the responsibility of respecting and serving the other. You are obligated to do so. Where art thou? Here I am! The students are moved by the painful plight of others. The students are taking a stand against those who fail to abide by another commandment emanating from the other's call of conscience: You shall not commit murder. The students are living for the other. It's a way of demonstrating and perfecting their goodness. In short, the students are showing Levinas how the utopian rapport with the other that his ethical philosophy requires can be put into practice. Levinas could not help being taken with all that went on in this dialogical situation.

Levinas, however, has nothing to say about how the actual conversation informed the dialogue: How did the students use language in evocative and interruptive ways to describe their reactions to the call of conscience? Did they argue and tell stories to make their particular points? Did they demonstrate considerateness and forbearance toward one another? Was their speech masterful, hyperbolic, inarticulate? If masterful, did it employ figures of thought and figures of speech to heighten one's consciousness and appreciation of the situation at hand and to sound the student's own call of conscience? These devices have long been recognized in the rhetorical tradition as forms of ornamentation that advance the perfectionist impulse of language to disclose the truth in heretofore unknown ways. This discursive practice defines the art of rhetorical eloquence. The seventeenth- and eighteen-century poet Fenelon speaks of the matter this way: Eloquence "is made up of the methods which reflection and experience have evolved to make a discourse such as to establish the truth and to arouse a love for it in the hearts of [human beings]. Things which strike and arouse the heart . . . eloquence is just that."[29] Eloquence is an agent for constructing narratives intended to cultivate wise judgment. Eloquence is acknowledged as a thing of beauty, and beauty can be seductive as it captivates the attention of its witnesses and serves as a model for improving their behavior. Eloquence is a way of facilitating wisdom and goodness. Eloquence lends itself to disclosing the truth. Kenneth Burke puts it this way: "The primary purpose of eloquence is to 'convert life' to its most thorough verbal equivalent."[30]

For Levinas, however, eloquence diminishes the saying of the primordial discourse of the face. Levinas associates the rhetorical workings of eloquence with "ruse, emprise, and exploitation." Elsewhere he claims that the practice of eloquence brings "into the meaning in which it culminates a certain beauty, a certain elevation, a certain nobility and an expressivity that imposes itself independently of its truth. Even more than verisimilitude, that beauty we call eloquence seduces the listener."[31] Levinas's one all-too-brief example is the media: "The media of information in all forms—written, spoken, visual—invade the home, keep people listening to an endless discourse, submit them to the seduction of a rhetoric that is only possible if it is eloquent and persuasive in portraying ideas and things too beautiful to be true."[32] With this example I believe Levinas is justified to associate eloquence with the use of beautiful language to seduce its listeners. The majority of corporate run media organizations are in the business of producing advertisement-soaked entertainment. Nevertheless, Levinas has an obsession with the negative that distorts his vision of the matter. I can use Levinas himself to make the point.

A religious individual, especially if he or she is Jewish, is likely to find Levinas's use of biblical references and the name of God throughout his writings to be captivating, beautiful, and seductive. His rhetoric heightens the individual's consciousness of the importance of transcendence and its spiritual grandeur. Levinas's rhetorical eloquence is undeniable. He converts the saying of the face into a said that speaks of unquestionable matters of importance. With his use of biblical references and the name of God—forms of ornamentation, to be sure—he finds a way to convert life into its most thorough verbal equivalent. It is an awesome accomplishment. Things which strike and arouse the heart . . . eloquence is just that. Yet, such accolades are not necessarily warranted. An individual who has the wherewithal to deal with Levinas's philosophy and who is an atheist is likely to find Levinas's use of ornate language to be a questionable, if not offensive, demonstration of rhetorical eloquence. It hardly is captivating, and its seductive beauty is a sham.

Levinas is not wrong in seeing beauty and seduction as being disturbing attributes of eloquence. But he is wrong to see these attributes as being but corrupting features of this rhetorical art. If only Levinas had admitted as much. The examples given help illustrate the confusion that results when the issue is not clarified. Perhaps he would have offered this clarification if he had been better educated in the teachings of the rhetorical tradition. Levinas does credit the interruptive call of conscience that comes from the face of the other and addresses the self as having a rhetorical impulse. In being addressed, the self, in turn, may have something to say. Now the other becomes the self. A philosophy of dialogue necessitates as much. The philosopher Hans-Georg Gadamer comments on the ethical nature of the conversation that should unfold as the self/other communicate with each other: "We say that we 'conduct' a conversation, but the more genuine a conversation is, the less its conduct lies within the will of either partner. Thus a genuine conversation is never the one we wanted to conduct. Rather, it is generally more correct to say that we fall into conversation, or even that we become involved in it. The way one word follows another, with the conversation taking its own twists and reaching its own conclusion, may well be conducted in some way, but the partners conversing are far less the leaders of it than the lead. No one knows in advance what will 'come out' of a conversation."[33]

Rhetoric facilitates this interpersonal interaction. The rhetoric of the self/other without another self/other makes no sense. As the philosopher Calvin Schrag points out, "The distinctive stamp of rhetorical intentionality is that it reaches out toward, aims at, is directed to the other as hearer, reader, and audience. This intentionality illustrates not the theoretical reflection of cognitive detachment but rather the practical engagement of concrete involvement. In the rhetorical situation the other is not set at a distance. He is 'engaged,' brought into the space of praxial concerns. The rhetor seeks to evoke from the hearer a response to a particular situation. He calls for deliberative action and reasoned judgment. . . . Rhetoric as the directedness of discourse to the other, soliciting a response, is destined to slide into ethics."[34]

What I am attempting to do is what Levinas does not do: demonstrate how the practice of rhetoric plays a significant role in cultivating the ethical relationship between the self and the other. The self has a moral obligation to serve the other. In a dialogue the self would have the right to be respected as another. Eloquence would help facilitate this exchange by enriching the dialogue's potential for maintaining the interests of each party and their commitment for generating a shared understanding of a given topic. And because things might not go smoothly as the self and the other conversed, the virtues of considerateness and forbearance acknowledged (although not practiced) by Heidegger would also be necessary. Indeed, thou shall not commit murder. If people are willing to develop their rhetorical competence so that they can better serve the other, then they first must assume the personal responsibility of deciding to do so. This requirement speaks of the importance of the self's authenticity. In being true to the interrupting call of the other, the self must also be true to the call of the interruption that we are. Levinas omits any consideration of this point. He assumed the personal responsibility of staying in the world of theory when advocating the ethical relationship that must exist between the self and the other. Theory needs practice to justify and, when necessary, refocus its vision. The process and results need not be pretty.

On September 16–18, 1982, Israeli-backed militants slaughtered more than several hundred Palestinians in the Sabra and Shatila refugee camp. The massacre was condemned worldwide. Levinas and the philosopher Alain Finkielkraut were invited to discuss the tragedy on Radio Communaute (September 28, 1982), hosted by the journalist Shlomo Malsa.[35] The rhetorical transaction was civil, focusing on Levinas's philosophy of the other and its relationship to political affairs. Near the end of the exchange, Malsa asked this question: "Emmanuel Levinas, you are the philosopher of the 'other'. Isn't history, isn't politics the very site of the encounter with the 'other', above all the Palestinian?" (294). Levinas's response was remarkable: "My definition of the other is completely different. The other is the neighbor, who is not necessarily kin, but who can be. And in this sense, if you're for the other, you're for the neighbor. But if your neighbor attacks another neighbor or treats him unjustly, what can you do? The alterity takes on another character, in alterity we can find an enemy, or at least then we are faced with the problems of knowing who is right and who is wrong, and who is just and who is unjust. There are people who are wrong" (294).

Levinas's response reflects a world of know-how whose narrative is unrelenting in speaking against another world of know-how (Palestinians and their backing by Hamas), whose narrative is equally unrelenting in commanding the annihilation of Israel. But Levinas's philosophy of the other is flawed in this rhetorical situation. The philosopher Slavoj Zizek offers a representative response to Levinas: "Levinas is basically saying that, as a principle, respect for alterity is unconditional (the highest sort of respect), but, when faced with a concrete other, one should nonetheless see if he is a friend or an enemy. In short, in practical politics, the respect for alterity strictly *means nothing*."[36] Practice trumps theory when theory fails to show its applicability to real-life circumstances. With its massacre of Palestinians, Israel is more of a Kierkegaardian and Heideggerian self than a Levinasian self. One demonstrates self-respect by assuming the responsibility of affirming his or her freedom through resolute choice. It's a matter of the self's authenticity.

Israel has been backed up against life and being for nearly four thousand years. The love of life has never ceased during this time. The interruption that we are has maintained its dual function and moral status. The health of the lived body is dependent on how well we deal with this fundamental interruption. A rhetorical narrative guiding the concerned thought and action of Israel is at work here and can be summed up in two words: "Never forget." The self wants to survive and demands respect. Tragically, massacres of the other happen. Indeed, practice trumps theory. The self need not serve the other to be a self that, in declaring the other to be "wrong" and ending the other's existence, maintains that he or she was behaving ethically.

I believe it would be extremely unwise to dismiss Levinas's philosophy because its creator failed to adhere to the dictates of his creation. If Heidegger's philosophy can be salvaged after what he did in 1933 and years after, then Levinas certainly deserves the same favor. I conclude this chapter with a brief case study that lends support to the value of Levinas's philosophy, although not without remaining concerned with the issue of the self's authenticity. The case is about the personal diary of Etty Hillesum, a twenty-nine-year-old victim of the Holocaust.

Etty Hillesum: An Interrupted Life

I never kept a personal diary, although I know a number of people who did and do. I've learned, although only in general terms, that people record all kind of things in their diaries: thoughts of the day, current experiences, wishes, fears, anxieties, dreams, love affairs, heartbreaks, hatreds, future plans, philosophical musings, suicidal thoughts, heroic expectations, and myriad other things. Day in and day out entries appear—a personal narrative in the making that brings some degree of order and sense to a self's life and that is meant only for the author's eyes. Privacy is sacred. Invasion by some other person is unethical, a grievous break of trust. The self is speaking to itself, not to the other. Of course, one can say, as does the philosopher Georges Gusdorf, that "Even in a soliloquy, in speaking to myself, I refer to myself as another. I communicate from myself to myself."[37] But that is not the other that Levinas is talking about. A personal diary is not in the service of the other outside oneself. The other need not be as sacred as Levinas would have it. A personal diary is a way for a self to be true to itself, to get itself together, to develop self-respect. Attempts to maintain the health of one's lived body should not be dismissed as being merely a selfish act. Levinas, of course, would be happier with the diarist if he or she created a narrative that better prepared the self to serve the needs of others (selves).

Etty Hillesum, born in Amsterdam in 1914, inhabited a cultivated world of know-how. Her father was a classical scholar. One brother was an accomplished pianist, the other a scientist. Hillesum received a degree in law and was a student of Slavic languages, philosophy, and psychology. She was known to have a vivid and caring personality, an active social life, and a penchant for bohemian lifestyles.[38] The ordering narrative of her world was interrupted as the anti-Semitism of National Socialism spread throughout Europe during the 1930s and the Nazi began occupying the Netherlands in 1942. The horror of the interruption and the narrative wreckage it caused exposed Hillesum to the interruption that we are, to that depth of existence that breeds anxiety and suffering, tests one's love of life, and encourages concerned thought and action. The interruption that we are functions simultaneously as a defeatist and a perfective force. Survival and sanity, the health of the lived body, requires that the self respond to the call of the interruption that we are. No matter how degrading it might be, a world of know-how that provides some semblance of order and meaning to the self's existence must be restored. The alternative is to perish in the narrative wreckage that now defines the self's fading life. The rhetorical construction of a narrative has a role to play in meeting the challenge at hand. Hillesum began writing her diary on March 9, 1941. The narrative continued until December 11, 1942. During this time, she volunteered to accompany Jews to a transit camp in Westerbork, where she worked in the camp hospital and was known as "the thinking heart of the barracks" (199). From Westerbork, the "detainees" were sent to Auschwitz. Etty was allowed to return to Amsterdam a number of times for brief visits. Eventually she, too, was shipped to Auschwitz.

Reading Etty's diary, one learns, as the author Eva Hoffman phrases it so well, that "Etty had the kind of genius for introspection that converts symptoms into significance and joins self-examination to philosophical investigation. The diary is a continuous, animated dialogue with herself, a constant drive toward her own truth" (viii). Given the gut-wrenching times when she decided to disclose this truth in her diary, alone in her small living quarters in Amsterdam, it is not surprising to find in her first entry (March 9, 1941) an admission: "So many inhibitions, so much fear of letting go, of allowing things to pour out of me, and yet that is what I must do if I am ever to give my life a reasonable and satisfactory purpose" (3). We are told this purpose as Etty writes about the development of the truth of her lived body—a truth that serves as a counternarrative to what the Nazi have in store for Jews. Etty prepared her mind for coming to terms with this truth by reading works of Dostoyevsky, Hegel, Rilke, and St. Augustine, whose *Confessions* (Latin: *confiteri:* to acknowledge) named the act that was needed to disclose the truth that Etty sought to reveal. The act is arduous but essential: "it's all a matter of looking for the right words," says Etty (13). The right words, the perfect words, show forth what something is. That's epideictic discourse. The right words, the perfect words help the self to convert life into its most thorough verbal equivalent. That's eloquence. Here is Etty employing both of these rhetorical phenomena as she discloses the difficulty of putting them to the best use:

> [T]here are . . . sudden bursts of creativity, but above all there is despair, so much despair at not being able to express any of the many vague and unclear things inside me. And finding that, though I'm getting quite old, I'm still without an "instrument" and without an "object." I must delve deep into myself and fetch up unformed slabs of granite and chisel them into shape. But no strength to lift them up as yet, no tool to hew the granite. . . . [A]t times I think that I will be able to write one day, to describe things, but then I suddenly grow tired and say to myself, "Why all these words?" I want every word I write to be born, truly born, none to be artificial, every one to be essential. For otherwise there is no point to it at all. And that is why I shall never be able to make a living by writing, why I must always have a job to earn my keep. Every word born of an inner necessity—writing must never be anything else. (118–19)

Etty has as her goal the rhetorical construction of a narrative that tells a story about herself and her circumstances. She is assuming the responsibility of affirming her freedom to create a world of know-how that is not mutilated by the narrative of National Socialism and its Nazi hordes. She is responding to a call from the interruption that we are. She is a self being true to herself. She is a self displaying her authenticity, her self-determination. Her evolving narrative is her own. She is Kierkegaard's "I." She is Heidegger's "Self." And as Etty gets closer to her inevitable fate and thus more caught up in the defeatist pull of the interruption that we are, she also becomes Levinas's self. Her concern for finding and cultivating the inner strength of herself becomes a concern for how well she can use that strength to serve others. Conscience calls: "Have I really made so much progress [in understanding my "self"] that I can say with complete honesty I hope that they send me to a labor camp so that I can do something for the sixteen-year-old girls who will also be going? And to reassure the distracted parents who are kept behind, saying, 'Don't worry, I'll look after your children'?" (171).

But notice the phrasing here. A self is going to place itself in the service of others. Yet it is a self that needs to reassure itself that she is ready to assume the ethical challenge. The other needs the service of a self that is experienced, competent, strong, wise, tested, prepared, and conditioned enough to do the job. The self has a lot of work to do before it can respond adequately, skillfully, honestly, wholeheartedly to the other's call of conscience. Etty agrees as she remains true to heeding another call: "Life is hard, but that is no bad thing. If one starts by taking one's own importance seriously, the rest follows. It is not morbid individualism to work on oneself" (145). And for Etty, the work must go on for as long as possible:

> When I tell others, fleeing or hiding is pointless, there is no escape, so let's just do what we can for others, it sounds too much like defeatism, like something I don't mean at all. I cannot find the right words either for that radiant feeling inside me, which encompasses but is untouched by all the suffering and all the violence. . . . We must learn to shoulder our common fate; everyone who seeks to save himself must surely realize that if he does not go another must take his place. As if it really mattered which of us goes. Ours is now a common destiny, and that is something we must not forget. . . . But I keep finding myself in prayer. And that is something I shall always be able to do, even in the smallest space: pray. . . . And I shall wield this slender fountain pen as if it were a hammer, and my words will have to be so many hammer strokes with which to beat out the story of our fate and of a piece of history as it is and never was before. (171–73)

The Nazi were torturing and killing her people. Eddy struggled to find the right words, the perfect words, to describe "the deadly fear . . . [she] saw in all those faces. All those faces, my God, those faces!" (184). The right words, the perfect words, were not always forthcoming. So she prayed some more: "Give me a small line of verse from time to time, oh God, and if I cannot write it down for lack of paper or light, then let me address it softly in the evening to your great Heaven. But please give me a small line of verse now and then" (215). And the prayers continued: Please God, "Let me be the thinking heart of these barracks" (225). Thinking heart. The right word. Etty prayed to God for that which could strengthen the health of her lived body and better prepare her as a self wanting to serve others: the right words to disclose the truth of her life and times. Her personal diary offers a narrative that tells the story of her struggle to accomplish the task. The diary offers evidence not only of the applicability of Levinas's philosophy but also how that philosophy needs amending regarding the character and rhetorical competence of a self desiring to do the best possible job in serving the other.

Etty turned down an opportunity to escape from Amsterdam; her calling was to remain in her hellish environment for the benefit of others. Her decision adds to the affirmation of the importance of Levinas's philosophy. And it also indicates the need for another amendment. Heschel makes us aware of what this amendment should be with the following observation regarding an essential feature of human existence: A self "insists not only on being satisfied but also on being able to satisfy, on *being a need* not only on *having needs.* Personal needs come and go, but one anxiety remains: *Am I needed*? There is not a man who has not been moved by that anxiety. . . . The feeling of futility that comes with the sense of being useless, of not being needed in the world, is the most common cause of psychoneurosis. The only way to avoid despair is to be a need rather than an end. *Happiness,* in fact, may be defined as the *certainty of being needed.*"[39]

Etty fulfilled this need by serving others who needed her, and she knew it. Knowing that you are needed and why that is so affects how you will serve the other. It is a very practical and concrete matter, which remains unaccounted for in Levinas's philosophy. More needs to be said about the self than is acknowledged by Levinas.

The amendments to his philosophy add to its relevance: The other offers a call of conscience that interrupts the self's existence such that the self owes allegiance to the other and is willing and able to fulfill this obligation. The accomplishment demonstrates an essential way that a self can abide by a Holy command: "Walk before me and be thou perfect." This is how the self lives a good life. Etty was involved in the activity up until the moment she was killed in Auschwitz. It may thus be said that in the end she was true to Levinas's philosophy. Indeed, Levinas has no reservations when he claims that "There is a responsibility for the other right up to dying for the other!"[40] The claim produces a paradox: The health of the lived body reaches perfection with this ultimate act of self-sacrifice. Levinas is defining what constitutes a good death for a self struggling to live a good life. He is being true to his religious heritage: "For the pious man," writes Rabbi Heschel, "it is a privilege to die."[41] With Levinas, we learn to associate the good life with specific virtues: morality, conscience, respect, and dignity. With Etty, the authenticity of self-determination, eloquence, and wholeheartedness are three additional virtues that warrant acknowledgment. The other is a powerful influence on the self's existence. The self is a powerful influence on the other's existence. The self is obligated to serve the other. The interruption that we are entails this moral obligation. Levinas's teachings are instructive, but they do not go far enough. The self is also obligated to serve itself so that it is better able to serve the other. The interruption that we are demands as much.

Before Etty was shipped to Auschwitz, she gave her diary to an associate who still lived in Amsterdam and requested that, if possible, arrangements be made to have the diary published if Etty did not return. A heartbreaking and inspiring narrative now answers the call of others who find themselves engaged in public moral argument regarding crimes against humanity. The Etty Hillesum Foundation keeps her spirit alive. We others need a self whose authenticity can serve us well. We need resolve, courage, strength, compassion, and narratives with the right words. Public moral argument requires rhetorically competent selves who, having served themselves by developing this competence, are better prepared to fulfill their obligation to serve others.

Over the years I have been critiqued by followers of Levinas for employing a host of his constructs to assess the practice of rhetoric in real-life cases of public moral argument. The critiques had a similar ring that sounded like this: "To evoke Levinas as a scholarly legitimization of actual communicative practices is to mislead the readers about Levinas and to twist his intent around into the opposite of what he meant. He is being hijacked." Indeed, Levinas's phenomenological analysis of the other and its relationship with the self is meant to describe the presuppositions of our everyday ways of being with others: How we exist before the social rules and routines of worlds of know-how conditions us to think and act in accordance with standards of common sense. We are exposed to others before we understand their needs; we are "hostage" to a "caress" of the other that chooses us before we decide to respond in any given case.[42] But with his stated claim about the self's responsibility to die for the other, Levinas is applying his philosophy to substantiate its real-life consequences. Selves (and others) die in the world of praxis, not in the world of theory. They die as they are contending with the interruption that we are, which, as Levinas helps us to understand, displays a moral function. I agree with Levinas's earlier quoted claim: "The Other becomes my neighbor [in the most communal and moral sense of the term] precisely through the way the face summons me, calls for me, begs for me [with its interrupting call of conscience], and in so doing recalls my responsibility and calls me into question." Highjacking this theoretical claim does not bother me a bit. Theory needs to prove its validity and value in the world of practice. Kierkegaard is worth repeating: "Existence constitutes the highest interest of the existing individual, and his interest in his existence constitutes his reality."[43] The interruption that we are makes itself known as we deal with everyday existence. This interruption is as real as real can be.

Summary

My reading of Kierkegaard, Heidegger, and Levinas on the interruption that we are helps to identify the intricacies of how this essential feature of human existence, with its defeatist and perfective impulses, influences the health of the lived body and calls for the rhetorical construction of narratives that can inform the communicative activity of public moral argument. Many additional and related topics warranted attention as I discussed these central concerns. There is a lot to say when attempting to tell a story about the nature, scope, and function of the interruption that we are, which shows itself as a rhetorical (epideictic) phenomenon. The dynamics of this interruption define an exceptionally powerful force of existence that can drive the self to its knees or encourage it to stay on its feet and act when faced with the trials and tribulations of life.

In the next four chapters I continue to offer case studies that focus on selves who constructed narratives that helped them deal with how their being exposed to the interruption that we are affected the health of their lived bodies and how these narratives were transformed into stories for the purpose of engaging in public moral argument about the selves' conditions. The first three stories form a progression of illness narratives that lead to a fourth story about the treatment of illnesses and the enhancement of the lived body's physical and mental capacities. Taken together, the stories encourage consideration of what constitutes the "good life." Recall, once again, that the interruption that we are can be read empirically as a gift of goodness. Goodness is perfection in the making. Goodness shows itself in virtuous behavior. Virtue is a character trait the humans must cultivate in order to flourish as a species and establish high quality relationships with others. The good life and virtue go hand in hand. Various virtues warranted consideration in my discussion of Kierkegaard, Heidegger, and Levinas. These virtues included wholeheartedness, self-determination, authenticity, the use of the perfectionist impulse of language to disclose the truth, acknowledgment, eloquence, considerateness, forbearance, listening, conscience, the self-other relationship, heroism, goodness, dignity, and moral integrity. All of these virtues play a role in the telling and progression of the stories.

The first story is told by Charles Siebert in his "The Rehumanization of the Human Heart: What Doctors Have Forgotten, Poets Have Always Known," which he revised and updated in his *A Man after His Own Heart.*[44] Siebert's story is about his heart ailment. As he talks about his illness, he recalls the plight of William Schroeder, the second recipient of the Jarvik-7 artificial heart, which could sustain the life of a patient whose own heart was failing and who was not young and fit enough to qualify for an actual heart transplant. Siebert's story is credited with offering "the most eloquent and poignant evocation of the emotional and existential capacities that many believed might have been taken from the Jarvik-7 recipients when their own hearts were removed."[45] The story makes a case for how the perfectionist use of language plays a role in establishing an emotional environment that is advantageous for maintaining the quality of doctor-patient communication, the social treatment of the patient, and the patient's psychological status. Medicine's concern with these matters dates back to the teachings of Hippocrates (5th century B.C.E.), the father of scientific medicine. Medicine is still struggling to deal with these matters in sufficient ways; hence, for example, the decision by the Association of American Medical Colleges in 2015 to add a "critical analysis/reasoning from the humanities" component to its Medical College Admissions Test (MCAT). For the purposes of my story, Siebert's story is ideal. I have yet to find a more original discussion, offered by a wounded storyteller engaged in public moral argument, of a patient's need to have the right words and narratives for coping with the emotional circumstances that arise when illness exposes him to the interruption that we are. In order to establish the necessary background for appreciating the full range of the story, I first offer some remarks regarding medicine's world of know-how. For here is where Siebert had the experience that prompted him to construct his narrative. These remarks will also be helpful for my discussion of the next two cases that inform my story. So, too, will this remark by the physician Eric J. Cassell: "Each of us gets to our illness our own way, it becomes part of our story, and we individualize it by its place in the narrative of our lives. To know that illness one must know something of the person. To know the person, one must know something of the narrative."[46]

CHAPTER 4

The Right Word

> "It is up to each person to assume the responsibility for his own language by searching for the *right word*."
>
> Georges Gusdorf, *Speaking (La Parole)*

I have never witnessed a physician give a formal presentation to an audience of his or her peers without slides. In today's computer age, the practice is commonplace in academic and business settings. For physicians, however, slides maintain an unequaled valuable status. Physicians have to see what a speaker is saying. They are trained as scientists, as hardcore empiricists. They need reliable data. They inhabit a world of know-how that is geared to prepare them to know everything they can about the disease in the body in the bed if they are to stand any chance to achieve their most rewarding goal: curing the patient's illness. That's perfection. Slides help condition physicians' senses. Slides show respect for proper protocol. Slides enhance the telling of a knowledgeable and respectable illness story. A physician mentor who helped me prepare for my first Grand Rounds lecture at a university hospital made sure I knew the rules: "You need slides. They need slides. Present them with slides. It is a perfect thing to do." A presentation to physicians that is not complemented with slides is an interruption. When trying to save the lives of their patients, physicians stand face to face with the interruption that we are.

As part of a field research project in health communication, I am attending morning rounds in an intensive care unit. The interns begin to report on the status of their patients. The reports are narratives in strict conformity with the rules of the interns' world of know-how. Here is an example: "63 y.o. male with past medical history significant for diabetes, hypertension, end stage renal disease with renal transplant in 2013, presented with clinical seizures and altered mental status. MRI was unremarkable for any acute intracranial abnormality. Lumbar puncture was done and cerebrospinal fluid analysis was done concerning for acute bacterial meningitis. Patient likely had seizure in the setting of meningitis.

Antibiotics were initiated. Patient is currently recuperating well with good response to antibiotics."

I have never heard a medical rounds report that did not contain the word "present" in its first sentence. The intern is giving a presentation of a presentation—one that demonstrates a disciplined use of the right words to disclose a disclosure: the patient's physiological condition. I have referred to the importance of this process previously in my story: Truth happens first and foremost as a disclosing of the world, a revealing of something that directs our attention. The intern needs to tell the true story of a disease, its pathophysiology. Her report is a verbal slide containing up to date diagnostic data. I heard my mentor's voice: "Present them with slides." Indeed, "the patient presented. . . ."

The intern is telling an illness story that involves two characters to whom things happen: a person and a person's body. The body has priority. Directed by this priority, the intern can tell a "body story" (as opposed to a "person story") that cuts like a scalpel through the personhood of the patient, thereby leaving intact only those portions of the patient's history that can be used to make a good case about some disease harming the health of a lived body. A body story is prized for its self-effacing objectivity and efficiency, both of which are registered via the antiseptic language of "disease theory" and what it has to say about such things as acute intracranial abnormality, lumbar puncture, and cerebrospinal fluid analysis.

Body stories and person stories are not meant to go together. They employ different language games. Their respective characters are incommensurate. They interrupt each other. Indeed, the idiosyncratic subjectivity of the person gets in the way of the scientific objectivity of the body. When this occurs, the medical matter at hand may become too time consuming, too existential, too uncertain and opinionated. The Hippocratic law long ago made it clear: "There are in fact two things, science and opinion; the former begets knowledge, the latter ignorance."[1] Body stories offer narratives that are law abiding.

Anyone who has ever benefited from a physician's ability to tell such a story may have little trouble testifying to its importance. Still, problems can and do arise when physicians' scientific conditioning and outlook blind them to the difference between physiology and the overall health of a lived body. What tends to be forgotten when such blindness occurs is that patients are also persons and should be treated as such. A diseased body is also a *lived* body that brings to the medical encounter a host of personal concerns, involvements, and values (a world of know-how) that the patient may want to have taken into account in designing a prescribed treatment regimen. Patients have the right to affirm who they are as lived bodies. It's a matter of self-determination. As the other interns take turns telling their body stories, I keep looking at a sign posted above the attending physician's head. I had read the sign many times before: "Do not treat the patients just by the numbers."

Every time I recall reading that sign, an expression comes to mind that indicates our perfectionist desire to find the truth about whatever concerns us: "Let's get to the heart of the matter." Heart and truth are known to coexist. Body stories must abide by the meaning of this expression. The relationship between the heart and truth is so significant that it is credited as being a gift from God. I quoted the relevant Scripture earlier: "I will give them a heart to know Me, that I am the Lord" (Jeremiah 24:7). There are two senses of "heart" at work here. To know the Lord (or any other matter of concern) requires that we think about Its truth: what, why, and how It is. To think about this truth also requires that one *care* enough to put forth the effort. To care about something is to form some emotional attachment to it. Having a heart for something enables us to feel and be moved (*emovere*) by whatever concerns us. Knowing and caring: That's why Etty prayed to God for a "thinking heart," which enabled her to grasp the horror of her situation, acquire self-understanding, feel for and serve others, and compose the narrative of her diary with the right words.

I am on call at night in the ICU. A young doctor, late twenties, walks into the room of an elderly male patient to report a battery of test results. The doctor calls the patient's name, gets his attention, looks concerned, and speaks: "Mr. Jones, we have the results from the tests and I am sorry to say that you do have cancer. The attending physician will be here shortly to talk to you about your situation." The doctor hesitated a moment, remained silent, and then walked out of the room and down the corridor. He did his job. He told the truth. It's the perfect thing to do. That's what counts when you have cancer. The disease in the body in the bed. The attending physician had a few "kind" words to share with his young colleague later that evening about the one-way brief transaction, which left the patient exposed, without a word, to the interruption that we are and that lacked considerateness and forbearance on the doctor's part. It was a startling interruption of the doctor's routine. The point was clear. There are other stories to be told, other stories to be listened to besides body stories. "What in the hell is wrong with you?" The doctor stood face to face with the interruption that we are and the obligation that it calls for: to acknowledge and serve others in a fitting way—one that allows them to have a say about their condition. The expression on the doctor's face said it all.

Don't treat the patients just by the numbers. This order assigns physicians the task of having a heart for the patient as person, as a lived body who has emotional needs that warrant consideration. Numbers and what they indicate are alone not enough. Illness brings a patient face to face with the interruption that we are, its defeatist and perfective impulses and its attending anxiety. The narrative of a body story is intended to interrupt this interruption by helping to provide a cure that can release the patient from the defeatist impulse of this interruption. The narrative of a person story can assist in the endeavor. The skill needed here is to listen to the stories that the patient has to offer and then respond in a fitting way. Remember, listening to others is the existential way of Being open to their assessment of the circumstances at hand. We are communal beings. The data acquired are qualitative. Another interruptive world of know-how is present and active. Comprehensive care of patients requires considerateness and forbearance in attending to the health of the lived body. Doctor-patient communication is a virtuous activity that involves people telling and listening to stories.

The literary critic Anatole Broyard addressed the matter shortly before he died from prostate cancer: "Always in emergencies we invent narratives. We describe what is happening, as if to confine the catastrophe. . . . Storytelling seems to be a natural reaction to illness. People bleed stories. . . . Stories are antibodies against illness and pain. . . . Anything is better than an awful silent suffering. . . . Stories can turn you off or turn you on." Broyard makes much of how a patient should try to tell an interesting story—one that might establish some emotional bond between the parties. Failing this, the patient's lived body invites insult. Many doctors "look at you panoramically. They don't see you in focus. They look all around you, and you are a figure in the ground. You are like one of those lonely figures in early landscape painting, a figure in the distance only to give scale. If he could gaze directly at the patient, the doctor's work would be more gratifying. Why bother with sick people, why try to save them, if they're not worth acknowledging. When a doctor refuses to acknowledge a patient, he is, in effect, abandoning him to his illness."[2]

Abandoning patients places them back face to face with the defeatist impulse of the interruption that we are. The patients are looking for a good audience that will acknowledge their struggle to align themselves with the perfective impulse of the interruption and create a redeeming narrative that will help them and their caregivers make total sense of the situation. If the patients are able to leave the hospital, the patients' stories might also serve others.

The sociologist Arthur Frank, whose work on narrative ethics is influenced by Levinas, makes much of the point: "People tell stories not just to work out their own changing identities, but also to guide others who will follow them."[3] Frank is specifically writing about what he terms the "wounded storyteller": a person who has suffered and survived the crisis of an illness and who is able to create a narrative that details the person's experience and that provides guidance for others who require help in dealing with their illness. "Ill people's storytelling is informed by a sense of responsibility to the commonsense world and represents one way of living for the other." The wounded storyteller "offers herself as a guide to the other's self-formation. The other's receipt of that guidance not only recognizes but *values* the teller. The moral genius of storytelling is that each, teller and listener, enters the space of the story *for* the other."[4] The teller and the listener engage in this act because they are *moved* to do so. Rhetorical competence facilitates this movement and the identification that is crucial for the self and the other to form some degree of kinship. It is a thoughtful, emotional, and educational experience. The teller and the listener have to have a thinking heart for each other. Frank writes: "In the beginning is an interruption. Disease interrupts a life, and illness then means living with perpetual interruption."[5] Indeed, coming face to face with the interruption that we are often leaves wounds that may never go away. Memories perhaps are here to stay. The work of a wounded storyteller is never done until her body story comes to an end. The heart stops, the brain dies. Yet even then the power of the teller's story may keep her life going, continuing to serve others in need. Worlds of know-how are always in demand. So, too, the praiseworthy rhetorical construction of narratives. People continue to read writers like Broyard for those very reasons. Have a heart. And the right word, too. Gusdorf speaks to this point: "The man of his word doesn't just give lip-service, but gives himself. . . . The great educator is he who spreads around himself the meaning of the honor of language as a concern for integrity in the relations with others and oneself."[6] The process helps people cultivate their rhetorical competence—the very thing that is needed to ensure the quality of public moral argument.

Charles Siebert

Gusdorf's advice provides an appropriate introduction to Siebert's article and book. Of the many things that were on Siebert's mind as he readied himself to write about the heart, the following two concerns are especially relevant for my purposes: "Where . . . to begin? At what point in the heart's motion, to intercede without disrupting that ongoing simultaneity? It has a mind of its own, the heart, for which our minds have yet to find the words" (M6). And later he says this:

> The closer [modern science] seems to bring us to the very essence of our and of all being, the less adequate words are for capturing that experience. It is as if, after all the mythic monsters and curses we have conjured over the centuries as the God-appointed guardians of ultimate truth—the fire-breathing dragons, the sudden earthquake fissures, the snake-filled pits, the skin-flaying potions, and so on, all those obstacles we've imagined coming between ourselves and the attainment of our myriad Holy Grails—the most formidable one, the one that the gods themselves, whoever they might be, have been putting the most stock in, is our own inarticulateness. (M125)

During an email exchange about setting up a phone interview to discuss his article and book, Siebert told me that his "article was in some ways aimed to rankle and rouse" physicians who showed little concern for how their scientific world of know-how and attending disciplined narratives of body stories dehumanized patients' lived bodies (May 20, 2016). Stimulating public moral argument was a goal. Responses to Siebert's story from the general public were positive. He had found the right words and was articulate. His rhetorical competence was praiseworthy. Physicians, on the other hand, displayed "outraged resistance." His words were not right. Rhetorical competence was lacking. He was articulate, but this skill only made the deficiencies more obvious. The diagnosis was easily discernible: Worlds of know-how and their narratives were interrupting each other. The proper use of the perfectionist impulse of language was a major matter of contention.

Siebert is a wounded storyteller. He suffered from a heart condition known as "heart hypochondria—a sudden, all-consuming awareness and fear of the very muscle that moves each of us, tentatively, from one breath to the next . . . [and that] is a fairly common phenomenon today, especially among my contemporaries, for whom that first late-night dash to the emergency room because of a skipped beat or a bad bout of indigestion is a kind of rite of passage, a first, close encounter with mortality" (R53). Siebert's heart problem started when he was twenty-two. He believed he "was dying from heart failure." He tells us that he "made three late-night visits to the emergency room in the same week for what this doctor had determined to be mere anxiety attacks." The interruption that we are is ever present. With the third visit the doctor grew impatient, "dragged" Siebert into the doctor's office, and explained "that he did have other patients with serious problems." The doctor "then picked up the plastic desktop model of a human heart before him and, with his pencil, poked at the various chambers and values—atrium, ventricle, mitral, and tricuspid," and then made his point: 'You see,' he said, 'a very efficient pump'" (R53).

Having heard similar stories from people over the years, Siebert came to a conclusion: "The consensus among physicians . . . [is] that the best way to cure this fear of one's heart is to instruct patients to look at the heart mechanically, technically—to, in a sense, dehumanize it. If the heart's a pump, there is nothing to worry about. We make those. They're simple, long-lasting, and easily repaired—even replaced, at least in part, when broken" (R53). A medical narrative was in control.

Siebert took exception to this mechanistic and reductionist view of the heart. He admits that he once was willing to accept its "gross oversimplification"; for, indeed, the "job" of physicians is "to mend and medicate hearts, not poeticize them." But now, given his medical problems, he realized he could no longer accept such common sense; for medicine's technological conception of the heart "has led to a diminished appreciation of the heart's subtleties and its spiritual relevance." According to Siebert, with the successes of our ever-growing biotechnological revolution "we may be suffering a kind of collective heart attack, a modern metaphysical one—pained by the weakening of long-held notions of the heart as the home of the soul and the seat of deep emotions" (R54). The vision of a posthuman future is present. Siebert points out that "we've grown accustomed to the image of the chest split open under operating room lights while a heart wall is mended, a valve replaced, or a quadruple bypass performed." He goes on to note, "We've seen the heart itself held aloft in a surgeon's hand, as it's passed from one dying person to another who might use it: A baboon heart being placed in a baby named Fae; and, just seven years ago, the implantation in a human body of a permanent artificial heart—the awful apotheosis of the pump, modern science's most presumptuous meddling yet with the mysteries of the human body" (R54). "Pump" is not the right word for a person story. It lacks eloquence. It's not the proper use of the perfectionist impulse of language. The patient (as other) needs a more caring response from a physician (as self). The self who has a heart for the other strengthens the emotional ties of the relationship by displaying compassion for the one who the self is obliged to serve. It is a dignified thing to do.[7]

Siebert's assessment of medicine is aligned with a narrative that is critical of the profession of medicine, began developing in the 1970s, and remains at work today. Dr. Ralph Crawshaw once put it this way: "By a curious inversion of human values, scientific-therapeutic zeal has become a new, iatrogenic disease, the technical fix. Caught up in the wonderment of our burgeoning technology, physicians become blind to the difference between physiology and life."[8] Although not concerned with medicine per se, Kenneth Burke, borrowing terms from John Dewey and Thorstein Veblen, offers a more nuanced way of diagnosing the problem haunting Siebert. The problem is a consequence of medicine's "technological psychosis." This is not to suggest that medicine is "mentally deranged" and that what it has come to be necessarily warrants condemnation. Burke does not use the word "psychosis" in the psychological sense. Rather, he employs it primarily to signify "a *pronounced character* of the mind" that instructs one's interests and occupations. The instruction can be so regimented that it conditions those who employ it to develop a "trained incapacity" to see beyond their disciplined ways of describing and appreciating as perfectly as possible the health of the lived body.[9] Allowing themselves to be totally dependent on the myopic nature of their language when conversing with patients, physicians may even warrant the accusation that they are being "rotten with perfection" in the administration of their duties. Burke's ways of stating the problem is noteworthy: "[E]ach of our scientific nomenclatures suggest its own special range of possible developments, with specialists vowed to carry out these terministic possibilities to the extent of their personal ability and technical resources. Each such specialty is like the situation of an author who has an idea for a novel, and who will never rest until he has completely embodied it in a book. . . . There is a kind of 'terministic compulsion' to carry out the implications of one's terminology."[10]

The way the young physician referred to earlier spoke to and behaved when interacting with the cancer patient is an example of being rotten with perfection. The lesson learned is invaluable: The perfective impulse of the interruption that we are can be taken too far in a person's life.

If I were Siebert's physician, heard all of this, and had the rhetorical competence to do so, I would offer the following reply: Although the quest for perfection can lead to disaster, not enough of this capacity can also be dangerous to one's health. Along with the ailment of being rotten with perfection, we must also take seriously the disease of being rotten with imperfection. This fact of life is given a humorous twist in an episode of the television comedy *Seinfeld* as the funny but irritating character George reflects on his "pathetic existence."

> Why did it all turn out like this for me? I had so much promise. I was personable, I was bright . . . oh, not academically speaking, but I was perceptive. I always know when someone's uncomfortable at a party. It all became very clear as I was sitting [alone] out there [on the pier] today. . . . Every decision I've ever made in my entire life has been wrong. My life is the complete opposite of everything I want it to be. Every instinct I have in every aspect of life, be it something to wear, something to eat . . . it's all been wrong. Every one. . . . I'm disturbed! I'm depressed! I'm inadequate! I got it all! And, yeah, I'm a great quitter. It's one of the few things I do well. I come from a long line of quitters. My father was a quitter, my grandfather was a quitter. . . . I was raised to give up.[11]

George is rotten with imperfection. His outlook toward the future is cynical and hopeless, uninformed by careful reasoning and lacking in moral responsibility. His character is not enriched by such attributes as intellect and ethics. That George is still able to feel bad about his situation is, however, an indication that a desire for perfection still flickers in his soul. Being rotten with imperfection is not a particularly praiseworthy way to be.

Patients with heart problems do not want their physicians to be quitters, rotten with imperfection; rather, they want them to have a perfect understanding of the heart's anatomy that goes far beyond what the physician showed in the office; hence medicine's perfectionist use of language: the heart chambers: atria and ventricles; the three layers of the heart wall: epicardium, myocardium, and endocardium; the heart's cardiac conduction made possible by the atrioventricular bundle, the atrioventricular node, purkinje fibers, and sinoatrial node; the heart's cardiac cycle: diastole phase and systole phase; the heart values: aortic, mitral, pulmonary, tricuspid; the heart's arteries: aorta, brachiocephalic artery, carotid arteries, common iliac arteries, coronary arteries, pulmonary artery, and subclavian arteries; the heart's veins: brachiocephalic veins, common iliac veins, pulmonary veins; and venae cavae. These are the terms one hears during medical rounds when physicians, abiding by the requirements of their world of know-how, are telling a body story about a patient's heart disease. The detail and precision are remarkable. It certainly is not an instance of being rotten with perfection, although it could be seen as such if the scientific terminology of the heart's anatomy were all that physicians used when consulting with their patients. In order to avoid this problem, physicians make it easy for patients to understand the anatomy of the heart. They call it a pump. To the extent that the patient has little or no understanding of this anatomy, the physician's use of the term is not a demonstration of being rotten with perfection. On the contrary, it is a reasonable way to serve the patient's need for information. Who doesn't know what a pump is?

I do not believe that Siebert would dismiss the good intentions of this rebuttal, but I feel certain that he would declare that it misses his point. A pump is a piece of equipment, a tool, a technology, a feat of engineering ingenuity. Beyond that, this machinery lacks little if any symbolic significance that is relevant to ascertaining the existential status of the health of the lived body. Matters would be different if, for example, the Bible reported that God said, "I will give them a pump to know me that I am the Lord." Then this mechanism would speak to us of our emotional capacity to be open to, acknowledge, know with, and have feelings for others. This capacity is not what the term "pump" brings to mind. One needs the heart to do that. Interpreted in the context of Scripture, this capacity is also associated with the goodness of our spiritual being. Demonstrating goodness in a wholehearted (recall the Hebrew term *tamin:* perfect) way is necessary if we are to abide by the command "Walk before me and be thou perfect." Goodness shows itself when we display heartfelt concern for people and creatures in need of help. Goodness is perfection in the making.

All that I am saying here need not be based on the Bible. The interruption that we are, with its perfective impulse, calls for all of this and more. The art of rhetoric (eloquence) helps establish our emotional attachments to things and others. It heightens our ability to reach people's hearts and move them toward the good. To repeat an earlier quoted teaching of Fenelon on eloquence: This way with words "is made up of the methods which reflection and experience have evolved to make a discourse such as to establish the truth and to arouse a love for it in the hearts of [human beings]. Things which strike and arouse the heart . . . eloquence is just that." A person who is heartless warrants scorn and condemnation. The history of the heart's symbolic meaning, to which religion and rhetoric contribute, confirms this judgment. The history is extensive. Using the Bible as our benchmark, this history is nearly 3,500 years old. The symbolic meaning of the heart informs a long-standing narrative about how caring and loving our species can be.[12] The language and teachings of this narrative are too easily forsaken when we think of the heart as a pump. Body stories favor the use of this mechanistic metaphor. Person stories favor a more heartfelt appreciation of the health of the lived body.

Siebert admits that what he is saying leads to the "shockingly unoriginal conclusion that the heart is the home of our emotions." For Siebert, however, the conclusion is nonetheless valuable for its instructive insight. Elaborating on the matter, Siebert says this: Behind the "lines of our most clichéd Hallmark Card phrases (my heartfelt joy or sympathy; my heart leaps, longs, aches, or breaks for you) there are physical correlatives, feelings in the body caused by or related to the varying actions of our heart." Importantly, he also notes "that over the centuries of thinking about and expressing our emotions, we've not arbitrarily assigned them to the heart but have been, in effect, trying to catch up, with language, to the physical sensations emanating from that part of our bodies when we feel something" (R55). A body story will speak of a "heart attack" (or, more properly, a "myocardial infarction"); a person story, what Siebert wants to tell with his rhetorical interruption of the rhetoric of body stories, has more to do with what the heart, the home of the emotions, has "to say" when illness wreaks havoc with the health of the lived body. Siebert tells us that he "got divorced from [his] heart" when first instructed to think of it as a pump. That he found the suggestion emotionally upsetting helps explain his use of the term "rehumanization" in the title of his essay. Divorces need not be permanent. Having a heart for one's one-time wife or husband can go a long way toward remedying the situation.

I have been told by physicians with whom I worked over the years that emotions can "get in the way" of their required scientific treatment of patients. The admission always brought to mind what Dr. Watson had to say about his friend the famous detective colleague Sherlock Holmes: He is "the most perfect reasoning and observing machine that the world has seen." His powers of observation and deduction are in great part due to his ability to halt the "intrusions" of emotion when doing his job. "Grit in a sensitive instrument, or a crack in one of his own high power lenses, would not be more disturbing than a strong emotion in a nature such as his."[13] The irony here is that for Holmes to be true to his investigative talents, he had to have a passion for dispassion. Holmes's stock in trade is nothing without the workings of emotion, which, as discussed earlier, enable us to take an interest in our environments, acknowledge the reality at hand, and know whatever we can about its being.

Siebert is as passionate about the heart as Holmes is about disclosing the indisputable facts of his cases. Siebert wants us to have a heart for the heart, to be open to and acknowledge something that is more than a piece of equipment, informs our humanity, and too often remains slighted in doctor-patient communication. (The problem continues today to haunt people's perception of physicians' communicative and rhetorical skills—their "bedside manner.")[14] The heart inspires and is inspired by virtues that play an important role in contributing to the quality of living a good life. Siebert is engaged in public moral argument about an issue that transcends the boundaries of the medical establishment. How often do you have a heart for others? What would life be like if no one acknowledged your existence? Let us think about the heart, Siebert suggests, as did the Spanish poet Vicente Aleixandre as he sought to know "if the heart is a rainstorm or a riverbank." Let us think about the heart as did Petronius in the *Satyricon* when, describing the sensation of fright, he coined the phrase "My heart was in my mouth" (56).

With all that he is telling us about the heart, Siebert is engaged in the rhetorical construction of a narrative that speaks to the status of the health of the lived body. Following his critical discussion of medicine's "demystification of the heart" with its use of the term "pump," Siebert continues constructing this narrative by offering additional detail about the first time he suffered heart problems. This move enhances the personal nature of his narrative, making what he has to say more interesting to readers because they can better relate to his story. Remember the rhetorical maxim: We interest people by dealing with their interests.

Siebert was at his parents' home recovering from a leg injury. His heart suddenly began a "frantic unraveling away from [him] at more than 200 beats a minute." The episode was a cause of great anxiety and crisis. He was face to face with the interruption that we are. The anxiety was overwhelming. He rushed to his parents, who were seated in the den. The journey was short, the memories long. His father had a bad heart. When his first attack happened, eleven years earlier, a clinician told his mother, "Your husband will be a vegetable for the rest of his life." His father suffered from "idiopathic hypertrophic cardiomyopathy," a gradual but relentless weakening of the heart muscle. The disease has no definite cause or cure and is believed to be congenital. Siebert was sure that he had his father's disease. Along with these recollections, Siebert also admits that, at the moment, his "own heart was . . . going out to [his father]—as if sympathy had a physical correlative" (55). The face speaks, and Siebert was open to what it had to say. He was a self who had served the other and he was also another who needed a self to serve him. Although he does not say so, I imagine Siebert's father's heart also went out to his son. Hearts have to break if they are to leave the body and go out to others. Heartbreak hurts. The pain is emotional, not physical, although emotional distress can cause physical ailments. If possible, think about what it was like when you were heartbroken. Why did it happen? How did you feel? Was it bad enough that, like some people I know, you "wanted to die"? Heartbreak can lead a person to succumb totally to the defeatist impulse of the interruption that we are.

Siebert uses the story of his father as a transition to another case that is filled with heartbreak and that is the focus to the second half of Siebert's story. The case is that of William Schroeder, who was the second man in history to receive a permanent, totally artificial heart (the Jarvik-7, named after the heart's designer, Dr. Robert Jarvik). The first recipient of this much-publicized biotechnological feat, Dr. Barney Clark (1921–1983), lived for 112 days, although his depression was so severe that "he asked to die or be killed" (59). Schroeder (1938–1986) lived for 620 days. He, too, suffered severe depression. Siebert does not report whether Schroeder made a similar request. I am unaware of any other source saying that he did. I am, however, old enough to recall the media circus that surrounded these cases and that celebrated how medical science and technology saved the lives of patients whose age and poor health status disqualified them from being candidates for a real heart transplant. In the midst of this circus was Schroeder, who had lost his heart to a pump and the external 230-pound, shopping cart–size machine that powered the Jarvik-7. Heath officials involved in the Jarvik-7 project and reporters made much of how Schroeder was a "brave pioneer setting off into unknown territory." He was a "hero," a man with a "lot of heart" (despite the fact that he had no heart). His bravery was equated with the journey of the U.S. Apollo astronauts. One NIH official who was interviewed by Renee Fox and Judith Swazey declared that "There's a mystique about the artificial heart. The artificial heart is a bit like a star on the flag, and stopping the artificial heart program would be like picking the star off the flag."[15] Schroeder was seriously ill, dying, and being *used* by the medical and political establishments to advance their narratives of scientific and nationalistic grandeur. Was this the self serving the other or the other serving the self? Levinas makes clear that the interruption that we are entails a moral imperative. The health of Schroeder's lived body attached to the Jarvik-7 makes one wonder about what was really going on here. Where was the heart in all of this?

Schroeder reported that he "felt restored and invigorated" with the Jarvik-7 pumping away. He had a congratulatory phone conversation with President Reagan. He was happy with his new heart, which "felt like 'an old-time threshin' machine" (R59–60). Siebert then tells us that eighteen days after the operation, Schroeder "suffered a devastating stroke that might have killed a man with a normal heart." The Jarvik-7, on the other hand, was "oblivious to the surrounding turmoil" and "continued vigorously pumping blood to the damaged area of the brain." The operation was, indeed, a success, but the outcome made the patient worse off. A significant ethical question would thus arise: "Considering the suffering Schroeder would endure afterward, did the Jarvik-7 enable him to make a supernatural recovery and deny him a natural death?" (R59). With Siebert's story in mind, it seems fair to say at the very least that the Jarvik-7 allowed Schroeder to experience a living death. The defeatist impulse of the interruption that we are was all too apparent.

Schroeder dealt with this agonizing situation as best as he could. But eventually there came a breaking point. Schroeder was losing his wits over his heart, "and for the most basic reason: the noise and the looming presence of his heart's drive machine, which, when he and his wife moved into the quiet, specially equipped apartment across the street from the hospital, became all too apparent, lording over their only private time together" (R6). Imagine what life would be like if every moment you were taking notice of your heart's workings. You would be like Siebert, who identifies with Schroeder, a man who admitted continuously that he "hated" his new heart. "Essentially, he could find no way to situate himself around a heart half outside him, could not grow accustomed to a stare and a noise he couldn't contain or quell, and was thus deprived of perhaps the most simple, individuating moment we have when, at rest, we curl up, involute, womb-ward, around our own heart's deep inner thrum" (R60). A hero, a man with a big heart, was losing his fight against the defeatist impulse of the interruption that we are. It was a heartbreaking situation. Remembering the good life was no longer worth the time.

Siebert elaborates on this situation by offering a description of an old magazine photo of the pioneer Schroeder. It's April 1985, five months after surgery. Schroeder sits in a wheelchair outside, waiting to begin a fishing trip with his family. "One son is pushing him up a hill, while a daughter walks along side with the book bag size portable heart driver over her shoulder and, in an upheld hand, the drive lines through which flows the air that powers her father's Jarvik-7 heart." Siebert notes that "Everyone is smiling eagerly for the camera," but not Schroeder. Rather, he "sits slumped forward and tilted to one side, his right hand tugging at his oversize t-shirt near where the drive lines enter through his stomach, his eyes fixed in a downward gaze." The presence, the face, of this person is not encouraging. "It's an unsettled posture, poised somewhere between protest and powerlessness, and his expression in truth can have no 'like,' no simile: It's the look of a man who has lost his heart." Owing to various physical problems associated with the operation (for example, acute kidney failure), Schroeder spent "much of the time in a twilight state," unable to say much about his heartless predicament. It's a lonely existence. The only "diary" he left contained "reams of technical data doctors collected through constant testing" (R57). A diary that's a body story, not a person story. Diary! A remarkable display of rhetorical competence. A wrong word is the right word to disclose the truth of an undignified situation. That's eloquence. I am confident Etty Hillesum would agree.

Siebert continues, setting up his eventual use of an earlier cited phrase taken from the historical narrative of the heart's symbolic meaning: "We know that Schroeder felt. He cried at his son's wedding . . . and cried continually over his predicament. But when a man's heart no longer works in concert with his feelings, does he lament that fact, and cry more? Having had his heart cut out of a lifelong internal conversation [with his brain], does he begin to dwell more exclusively in his brain; to draw, in computer-like fashion, on a memory of his old heart's role in the emotional equation; and to proceed toward a realm for which there is no human precedent: a man whose heart is all riverbank and no rainstorm?" (59).

That is not all what the heart is supposed to be. In moments of immense joy and tremendous grief, the heart overflows its banks. It is a natural, normal, and healthy thing to do.

Siebert tells us that "Dr. Jarvik wrote of his own invention that its ultimate test would be whether it was 'forgettable.'" Indeed, as discussed in chapter 2 when we were assessing, with Heidegger's help, how worlds of know-how work, a good technology is one that is so transparent that it disappears before one's eyes and other sense organs. The good life entails becoming accustomed to life's interruptions, at least to the extent that their presence poses no significant challenge to our feeling good. Siebert ends his person story by describing a "chilling" episode that Schroeder had with his wife shortly before he died. The pump was in the way, more noticeable than ever. "[B]arely able to speak because of a stroke, [Schroeder] tried to signal to his wife from whatever place it was the Jarvik-7 had taken him to. He'd point to himself and then to her, to the heart-drive machine alongside him, and then to the empty space beside her. He kept repeating the signals and asking, 'Why?' Confused at first, his wife eventually asked him if he meant he wanted her to have a heart machine too. Schroeder, nodding vigorously, said, 'Yes'" (60).

I find this ending intriguing. Apparently, Schroeder wanted to be closer to his wife as he was dying. He wanted them to feel and know together. A final chance for a truly heartfelt moment of immeasurable love. Schroeder was a self who could no longer serve the other. Rather, he was an other in desperate need of a self willing to answer his call and acknowledge what was left of his humanity. The challenge for the wife was to submit to a mechanized and sufferable way of existing—one that would likely lead to her own death. The face speaks. The other interrupts the self. Levinas insists that "There is responsibility for the other right up to dying for the other."[16] The wife could see the pump, hear the pump, watch it control her husband's fading lived body. There was nothing pleasant going on here. It was heartbreaking. Did Schroeder really mean that he wanted his wife to have a heart machine? Was that a selfish request, inspired by love? Heroes are not selfish souls. I wanted to know what the wife said after Schroeder said "yes." I wanted to see an attempt at being rhetorically competent. The interruption that we are calls for open-mindedness, acknowledgment, a knowing-with others, and the rhetorical competence that is needed to bring about and advance this communal bonding and to disclose the truth in a moving way. How did the wife respond to this call? Questions are interruptions. Public moral argument is an interruption that can stimulate a desire to know more about the matter at hand. After reading Siebert's story, I wanted to know more. Have a heart, Siebert! Is leaving a story unfinished a mark of rhetorical competence, of caring for your audience? It is if the author believes that he has told a story that is good enough to keep the reader's interest, to incite the reader's inquisitiveness, and if the author trusts the reader's ability to keep the conversation going by acquiring additional information that may add some degree of completion to the author's rhetorical construction of his narrative. In public moral argument, the self serves the other. Now the roles are reversed.

The headstone marking Schroeder's grave is made of black granite in the shape of two overlapping hearts. One is laser engraved with an image of the Jarvik-7.[17] Apparently Schroeder's family was exceptionally grateful for what Dr. Jarvik and his pump had done for their heroic loved one. But public response lent a cautionary note. For example, Dr. Rivers Singleton Jr., a research scientist who spent more than twenty years pursuing questions about living organisms and who followed the developments of Schroeder's ordeal, had this to say about Jarvik's treatment of his hero:

> To my mind, a hero is a person who invokes inspiration in my life. A hero calls to mind high values that transcend and enrich my life. A hero provides insights into the capacity for human existence that go beyond my daily experience. For these reasons, I cannot envision Mr. Schroeder as a hero. By this I do not mean to expunge his memory or denigrate his suffering. His memory in the annals of humanity is important, and his suffering was great. To my mind, however, Mr. Schroeder was more victim than a hero. Mr. Schroeder was a victim of a philosophy of medicine that places the presence of life above the quality of life, a philosophy that values technology more than humanity. Mr. Schroeder's humanity was replaced by the existence of an experimental animal. He in essence became a guinea pig. (It is important to note the absence of the adjective human in that sentence.)[18]

Put another way, Jarvik and his colleagues were rotten with perfection. The hero narrative diverted attention from this sad state of affairs. Siebert's story is a rhetorical construction of another narrative meant to correct this wrong.

Singleton later emphasizes in his letter that he was not suggesting that human experimentation should cease. "If science is to continue improving the lot of humankind, experiments involving human beings must be performed." Indeed, Clark and Schroeder volunteered for their procedures. But it is clear that Singleton wanted the medical profession to have more of a heart for patients, especially those involved in research experiments. The importance of the request was undeniable when the research investigators Renee Fox and Judith Swazey, conducting interviews in the early 1990s with personnel responsible for assessing the ethical issues associated with Jarvik's pump, discovered inexcusable behavior. The investigators found that "most of those with grave doubts about the artificial heart experiment, who might have altered its course, remained silent and inactive despite their concerns." The practice "is a familiar, recurrent, socially predictable pattern in medicine. . . . Integral to this pattern is the shared belief that individuals will regulate themselves regarding standards of professional competence and conduct, as well as the norms of loyalty to the group that foster a collective self-protectiveness." Moreover, physicians "are disinclined to openly challenge, much less stop, research they find scientifically and ethically dubious." In January 1990, the Food and Drug Administration issued a recall of the Jarvik-7. Rotten with perfection, indeed. The perfective impulse of the interruption that we are was out of control. Internal Review Boards would never be the same.[19]

What is missing in Siebert's story further confirms its importance. Siebert has a heart for the heart. He believes that this feeling is a testimony to human dignity; it thereby should not be diminished, taken for granted, and forgotten because of the power of a medical rhetoric that certainly serves a legitimate purpose. We need pumps, and we need hearts. We need body stories, and we need person stories. Body stories display a passion for dispassion. Person stories display a passion for compassion. Siebert's story is a case in point. He answers the call of the interruption that we are. He makes good use of the perfectionist impulse of language. The right words appear throughout his story, informed by the historical narrative of the heart's symbolic meaning. These words moved this reader to have a heart for what their author had to say. A lesson in rhetorical competence is at hand. Public moral argument is an emotional endeavor, with potential consequences for the health of the lived body. Siebert is well aware of this fact. He had to be, given his topic and all he had to say about it.

On September 6, 2006, the U.S. Food and Drug Administration (FDA) approved the first totally implanted artificial heart. Created by AlcoMed Systems, the technology was designed for patients who were not eligible for a heart transplant and who were unlikely to live more than a month without intervention. The technology consisted of a two-pound internal battery mechanical heart that took over the pumping function of the diseased heart, which was removed during the implantation procedure. The battery allowed the recipient to be free from all external connections for up to one hour. Then the battery had to be recharged by an external battery. Unlike the Jarvik-7, patients were not tethered to a large and noisy air-pumping console.[20] The technology's size and placement inside the body made it more transparent, but its use was still mechanical—a pumping device. Due to insufficient evidence of its efficacy, AlcoMed abandoned further development of the product in 2014. Progress would, however, continue. Improvements in the mechanical design of artificial hearts by such companies as SymCardia Systems, have led to a decrease in recipients' morbidity and mortality rates.[21] Pumps have great value. Still, the emotional stress associated with receiving an artificial heart remains high. Siebert saw it coming. And there is a lesson to behold: when interruptions expose us to the interruption that we are, this essential feature of existence is sure to remind us that the heart, as it overflows its banks, is something more than a pump.

CHAPTER 5

The Self as Other, the Other as Self

"It takes a self to evoke a self."

Henry W. Johnstone Jr., *The Problem of the Self*

As I was finishing up a draft of the preceding chapter, I was invited to attend a workshop on doctor-patient communication in interview consultations, to be held at a medical school of a major university research hospital. Listening to what the physicians were teaching their colleagues about the topic and watching them engage in role-playing situations, I had no doubt that Siebert's story would be invaluable for their purposes. The story is unique in teaching physicians about the importance of the relationship between emotion and the health of the lived body. With both the workshop and my book stimulating my thoughts, I decided once again to contact Siebert (June 10, 2016) to chat about the heart and to ask him a question: "Are you still disabled by your illness?" My phrasing of the question was strategic. I had the present chapter in mind. He replied: "No, I no longer suffer from heart hypochondria. Slew that dragon in increments. . . . And yes, I think that kind of hypochondria can become quite disabling and depressing."

All illnesses, be they physical or mental, give rise to various degrees of disability and possibly depression. Siebert was able to deal with his illness and overcome its effects. The perfective impulse of the interruption that we are worked to his advantage, preventing him from being continually victimized by the defeatist impulse of the interruption. The severity of Schroeder's illness, disability, and depression were too incapacitating and destructive to remedy. Nobody in his or her right mind would want to live and die as he did. This reaction to Schroeder's condition can also occur when people are disturbed by the disabilities of others whose illnesses are not life-ending but are crippling enough to make people cringe at the thought that the health of their lived bodies could turn that pitiful.

Individuals with these disabilities know what it means to come face to face with the interruption that we are. Reactions to their presence can keep them in that state of being.[1]

People with traumatizing disabilities are not by commonsense definition "pictures of health." Challenging and changing this definition is crucial if the disabled are to maintain their integrity, self-respect, and psychological well-being. Finding the right words is essential. When one's body breaks down or is otherwise disabled and is exposed to the interruption that we are, it sounds a call of conscience. The broken body is an interruption to itself as well as to others; it presents discomfort to those who must live with it and to those who witness its dysfunction. Consider, for example, the physical disabilities of people whose arms and legs no longer work or are gone completely and whose existence depends on such things as hard-to-take drugs (such as chemotherapy), wheelchairs, ventilators, respirators, dialysis machines, artificial hearts, and similar types of medical technology. Can I live on? Would I want to live on? These are the basic questions that are typically raised as illness and accident wreak havoc with our bodies and thereby show the world a face that can tell with much practical wisdom a story of life and death, a story that reminds us that as soon as you are born you are old enough to die.

Arthur Frank notes that "one of our most difficult duties as human beings is to listen to the voices of those who suffer. The voices of the ill are easy to ignore, because these voices are often faltering in tone and mixed in message, particularly . . . before some editor has rendered them fit for reading by the healthy. These voices bespeak conditions of embodiment that most of us would rather forget our own vulnerability to." Frank admits that listening carefully to these voices is hard, but, like the telling of stories, it too is "a fundamental moral act."[2] The voices of the disabled make clear that they are not ready to give in to the defeatist impulse of the interruption that we are, that they are not ready to die. Still, ill-conditioned reactions to their presence can further damage the health of their lived bodies. Not being totally open to the disabled not only helps people avoid offering such reactions (which promote social death) but also makes it easier for them to ignore their own mortality and to avoid the anxiety that can accompany thinking about their inevitable fate of decline, decay, and unattractiveness.

There is something strange going on here. People are being polite to others by closing themselves off to the pains, sufferings, and needs of those others. Where art thou? The response of Here I am! in this situation is too half-hearted, selfish, and protective of the self rather than the other. The disabled lack genuine acknowledgment from those who can hear their call—"Thou shalt not commit murder"—and who thereby have a responsibility to respond to it. A world of know-how exists that says that it is acceptable to quit trying to be more than polite to the disabled, to those who are other than "normal" human beings. Quitters, we have seen, invite the characterization of being rotten with imperfection. Diane Coleman, a disability rights activist and the founder of the disability rights organization Not Dead Yet, suggests that this characterization may be too kind. According to Coleman, "There is a great revulsion against disabled people that is visceral. This disdain is masked as compassion but many people believe that in an ideal world, disabled people wouldn't be there."[3] An ideal world defines an environment that is as perfect as it can be. Disabled people embody imperfection. They thus are disqualified from being members of an ideal world. Their absence from this world would free people from having to deal with an imperfection that is disabling to others. Ridding an ideal world of disabled people is a perfect thing to do. Taken to its extreme, such a cleansing action defines a procedure named eugenics. Recall that, as recorded in the Bible, God practiced eugenics to eliminate evil. Recall, too, that eugenics was favored by Hitler. More people associate eugenics with Hitler than with God. And Hitler's attempt to create an ideal world demonstrated the horror of a disease: being rotten with perfection. The disability community is engaged in a continuous struggle to control, if not eliminate, this disease. Coleman has this disease in mind when speaking about the "disdain" that people have for disabled people. The philosopher Friedrich Nietzsche heightens this disease to sickening levels in his "A moral code for physicians": "The invalid is a parasite on society. In a certain state it is indecent to go on living. . . . When one *does away with* oneself one does the most estimable thing possible: one thereby almost deserves to live . . . one has freed others from having to endure one's sight, one has removed an *objection* from life."[4]

Adding to this problem is a related issue that is evident in the debates that disability rights activists have with those who support the "right to die" and physician-assisted suicide. Advocates of the right to die often advance arguments by telling stories of pain and suffering that people with disabilities know all too well but that are now being employed for the specific purpose of having people realize that they have the right *not* to live that way. This added burden is ethically and rhetorically significant. The disabled who want to live on are made to listen to discourse that uses the material of their lives to justify why people who suffer as they do need not and should not be forced to live on. The disabled thus find themselves in a situation where their own existence, which has already been marginalized by society, is now actually being turned against them by people whose stories and arguments, ironically, are meant to ease the pain and suffering of people with disabilities.

Disability rights activists dedicate themselves to securing and advancing the health of the lived bodies of disabled people. Offensive ways of thinking about and treating these people must be changed. Indeed, the right words are not being used. Having a heart for the disabled is shamefully perfunctory. Societal conditions must be conducive to encouraging the disabled to make use of the perfective impulse of the interruption that we are and thereby enact their authenticity, their self-determination to maintain and enhance their status as dignified individuals warranting genuine respect. Wholeheartedness, authenticity, self-determination, dignity, and respect are virtues needed to cultivate the moral character of human beings. The disabled are selves who are too easily "othered" and marginalized by people who have a hard time dealing with those whose disabilities constantly expose them to our interruptive nature. The face speaks: Thou shall not commit murder. The disabled are well aware how easy it is to ignore this command.

The self as other, the other as self: The disabled are engaged in a constant struggle to make this transformation a long-lasting reality. Rhetoric can help the disabled achieve this goal. As the philosopher and intellectual historian Hans Blumenberg notes: "Rhetoric is a system not only of soliciting mandates for action but also of putting into effect and defending, both with oneself and before others, a self-conception that is in the process of formation or has been formed."[5]

Harriet McBryde Johnson

Harriet McBryde Johnson was an attorney and a highly regarded disability rights activist associated with Not Dead Yet. She was born with a degenerative neuromuscular disease and confined for life to a wheelchair until she died, in 2008, at the age of fifty. Peter Singer, a professor at Princeton University, is well known for his strong support of animal rights, the environment, and the poor and needy, and for his unflinching advocacy of euthanasia for infants with severe disabilities. His guiding philosophical orientation is that of "Preference Utilitarianism," which "holds that we should do what, on balance, furthers the preferences of those affected" and which defines "a straightforward ethical theory that requires minimal metaphysical presuppositions [for example, a belief in God]."[6] The disability community sees this philosophy's support of euthanasia as a catalyst for spreading the disease of being rotten with perfection. Members of this community might not be alive today if Singer's philosophy were the established societal norm when they were infants. Their lives might even have ended in the womb, where their inevitable imperfections were first diagnosed.

Singer invited Johnson to Princeton to give two presentations that would serve as the basis for discussing their radically different perspectives on the treatment of infants with severe disabilities. The first, offered to 150 undergraduates, was on the eugenic practice of selective infanticide; the second, held during a dinner for Johnson, was on assisted suicide. Arguments were inevitable, at least between Johnson and Singer—between an other and a self whose arguments would challenge the other to demonstrate the authenticity of self-determination and the skill of rhetorical competence in order to articulate cogent and convincing counterarguments. The quotation from the philosopher and argumentation theorist Henry Johnstone Jr. that introduces this chapter offers an abbreviated description of this situation: "It takes a self to evoke a self." The existential features of the situation are worth noting. These features emerge as the arguers, committed to disclosing the truth of the matters at hand, maintain an open-minded attitude to counterarguments and thereby assume the risk of having to admit that their current understanding of these matters is deficient. Johnstone puts it this way: The "risk a person takes by listening to an argument is that he may have to change himself. . . . An arguer who wants control pure and simple does not argue; he controls by nonargumentative means and avoids risk. . . . To argue, a person must maintain the tension between control and what limits control. This tension may be characterized as tolerance, intellectual generosity, or respect."[7] Considerateness, forbearance, dignity, and moral integrity also facilitate this needed tension. At its best, argumentation is a virtuous activity called for by the interruption that we are. And this being so, Johnstone would have us realize that "argument is a defining feature of the human situation. A being not capable of arguing or of listening to argument would simply not be human. Such a being would lack a self."[8]

The world of argumentation is a world of know-how, which awaited Johnson as she headed to Princeton. In her *New York Times Magazine* article "Unspeakable Conversations," Johnson tells a story about her life and thoughts before, during, and after her interactions with Singer, students, and other interested parties in this world of know-how.[9] These interactions were the catalyst for writing the story, considered a classic in the disability rights literature on the use of public moral argument to clarify, justify, and defend these rights. What Johnson tells us in her story remains relevant today. The health of those like Johnson, with their imperfect lived bodies, is still jeopardized by the injurious ways that people think about and act toward the disabled. Current websites for the disability rights group Not Dead Yet make that clear.[10] I feel certain that Siebert would favor what Johnson has to say. Her story affirms the importance of genuinely having a heart for others who warrant the utmost respect for their praiseworthy efforts to live a good life.

"Unspeakable Conversations": an oxymoron, a rhetorical interruption, created by an imperfection, a living interruption, a wounded storyteller who describes herself as "the token cripple with an opposing view" (1). This storyteller makes use of the perfectionist impulse of language to construct a narrative whose rhetoric is intended to interrupt another narrative that is interrupting the health of a lived body and exposing it to what an illness has already exposed it to: the interruption that we are. I suspect that the title of Johnson's essay, like any strategic use of interruption—Kierkegaard's art of communication comes to mind—is meant to give us pause for thought, to have us wonder about and stay open to what directs our attention. Johnson maintains this inquisitive state as she begins her story, leaving unidentified who she is talking about. What she has to say increases our desire to discover who this person is, although if you know where Johnson is coming from the initial wonder subsides: "He insists that he doesn't want to kill me. He simply thinks it would have been better, all things considered, to have given my parents the option of killing the baby I once was, and to let other parents kill similar babies as they come along and thereby avoid the suffering that comes with lives like mine and satisfy the reasonable preferences of parents for a different kind of child. It has nothing to do with me. I should not feel threatened. Whenever I try to wrap my head around his tight string of syllogisms, my brain gets so fried it's . . . almost fun. Mercy! It's like 'Alice in Wonderland'" (1).

These last two sentences reflect a jocular rhetorical style that punctuates portions of Johnson's story and that contrasts with moments of her being dead serious when sharing her disgust for Singer's philosophy. The contrast makes the jocularity and seriousness more striking and evocative. Georges Gusdorf speaks of "the ceaseless heroism necessary in pursuing the struggle for style"—a struggle whereby "concern for the right expression is bound up with concern for true reality: accuracy (*justesse*) and integrity (*justice*) are two related virtues." For Gusdorf, the importance of style cannot be overemphasized: "Each of us, even the most simple of mortals, is charged with finding the expression to fit his situation. Each of us is charged with realizing himself in a language, a personal echo of the language of all which represents his contribution to the human world. The struggle for style is the struggle for consciousness (*la vie spirituelle*)."[11]

Johnson is engaged in a struggle for style that reflects her personality. She is a "real character," not a rule-following debater. And for her present purposes that demeanor is quite fitting. The rhetorical competence that informs public moral argument need not be as formal as it is expected to be in an official academic or political debate. The audience at Princeton is different from the audience that reads Johnson's story in *The New York Times Magazine*. The interests, training, and demands of these audiences are not the same, and these differences need to be taken into account when constructing what the rhetor hopes is an effective narrative for general public consumption.

Following the moment of jocularity, Johnson identifies "He" as Professor Peter Singer, "often called—and not just by his book publisher—the most influential philosopher of his time. He is the man who wants me dead." Johnson then immediately admits that this last claim is "not at all fair." A clarification is thus needed. The one she offers expands on what she said when beginning her story and, in so doing, provides a more detailed account of Singer's philosophy:

> He wants to legalize the killing of certain babies who might come to be like me if allowed to live. He also says he believes that it should be lawful under some circumstances to kill, at any age, individuals with cognitive impairments so severe that he doesn't consider them "persons." What does it mean to be a person? Awareness of your own existence in time. The capacity to harbor preferences as to the future, including the preference for continuing to live. At this stage of my life, I am a person. However, as an infant, I wasn't. I, like all humans, was born without self-awareness. And eventually, assuming my brain finally gets so fried that I fall into that wonderland where self and other and present and past and future blur into one boundless, formless all or nothing, then I'll lose my personhood and therefore my right to life. Then, he says, my family and doctors might put me out of my misery, or out of my bliss and oblivion, and no one count it murder. (1)

I consider what Johnson is saying to be a fair summary of Singer's position on eugenics and euthanasia. I will have more to say about this position shortly. For the time being, however, I stay with Johnson.

When I show students pictures of Johnson, even if they have already found them on the Internet, they respond with pained looks. Another common response is "Oh my God." Johnson would smile. She is an atheist. Making the best use of the perfective impulse of the interruption that we are is totally up to her. The defeatist impulse of the interruption is her enemy. She is not a quitter. She is not rotten with imperfection. It is wise to stay out of her way as she makes that clear. For example, she is (in)famous for loudly opposing "the charity mentality" and "pity-based tactics" of the annual Jerry Lewis muscular dystrophy telethon. And she firmly and consistently held her ground as Lewis made clear that he had no intention of ever making peace with opponents such as Johnson. He likened the idea of meeting with them to entertaining Hezbollah or insurgents in Iraq.[12] The students are inspired by her self-determination, especially given her physical impairment, which they find haunting. Johnson has seen this emotional reaction far too many times. Her story contains an example of how she responds: "It's not that I'm ugly. It's more that most people don't know how to look at me. The sight of me is routinely discombobulating. The power wheelchair is enough to inspire gawking, but that is the least of it. Much more impressive is the impact on my body of more than four decades of a muscle-wasting disease. At this stage of my life, I'm Karen Carpenter thin, flesh mostly vanished, a jumble of bones in a floppy bag of skin."

Johnson goes on to note that in childhood she was fitted for a back brace but decided at fifteen years old to throw it away and let her spine "reshape itself into a deep twisty S-curve. Now my right side is two deep canyons. To keep myself upright, I lean forward, rest my rib cage on my lap, plant my elbows beside my knees. Since my backbone found its own natural shape, I've been entirely comfortable in my skin. I am in the first generation to survive to such decrepitude. Because antibiotics were available, we didn't die from the childhood pneumonias that often come with weakened respiratory systems. I guess it is natural enough that most people don't know what to make of us" (2).

Johnson is educating us about her history, the posture of her lived body's everyday existence, and the inadequacy of people's perception of her. The difficulty of dealing with the inadequacy is illustrated and emphasized by Johnson's rhetorical maneuver of using self-deprecating humor to characterize the Karen Carpenter–like features of her lived body. All of this education is offered before she begins telling the story of her experience at Princeton. The education is necessary if the experience is to be fully appreciated. An earlier quoted insight shared by Eric Cassell is worth recalling: "Each of us gets to our illness our own way, it becomes part of our story, and we individualize it by its place in the narrative of our lives. To know that illness one must know something of the person. To know the person, one must know something of the narrative."[13] Johnson wants us to know all of this. And a bit more education is needed. She focuses on the way people see and react to her presence.

When she is out in public, people are moved to comment: "I admire you for being out; most people would give up"; and "God bless you! I'll pray for you"; and "You don't let the pain hold you back, do you?"; and "If I had to live like you, I think I'd kill myself" (2). Such comments reflect the conformist nature of a world of know-how where the perfectionist use of language is dull and uneducated when it comes to disclosing the truth of people like Johnson. The interruption that we are calls for openness, acknowledgment, community, and the disclosing and evocative power of eloquence. Johnson is telling a story that seeks to have people hear and respond to this call. She is an interruption exposing people to the interruption that we are and its perfective impulse. People can do better than telling her that they would kill themselves rather than be like her. Johnson writes: "I used to try to explain that in fact I enjoy my life . . . that I have no more reason to kill myself than most people. But it gets tedious." Worlds of know-how can condition their inhabitants to have a shallow understanding of what it means to have a heart. Johnson continues: "God didn't put me on this street to provide disability awareness training to the likes of them. In fact, no god put anyone anywhere for any reason, if you want to know. [So much for Kierkegaard.] But they don't want to know. They think they know everything there is to know, just by looking at me. That's how stereotypes work. They don't know that they're confused, that they're really expressing the discombobulation that comes in my wake" (2).

The virtues of considerateness and forbearance can fade fast when others who are part of your everyday existence fail to put into practice what the interruption that we are calls them to do. The problem here is a perfect example of the deficiency of Levinas's ethical philosophy of the other. The self is obligated to serve the other. Johnson is an other. Although exceptions exist, this other is served by kind comments from selves. But these selves are so lacking in interpersonal and rhetorical competence that their service proves antiproductive. Johnson demands respect, wholehearted acknowledgment. Anything less adds to the difficulty of trying to live a good life.

Johnson is telling a story that is motivated by her illness and reactions to it. The story is a major part of the narrative of her life. As we learn about her illness, we come to know significant aspects of her personhood, which in turn helps us better understand the narrative. Johnson is cognizant of the need to be rhetorically competent in facilitating this process. Elsewhere she writes: "My professional and political life is all about using words to influence behavior. Persuading people requires conveying information, surely, but also eliciting emotions. Whether I'm writing a legal brief for a judge, an eye-catching press release or broadside, or a short letter to a semi-literate client, the basic challenge is the same."[14] And meeting this challenge is aided by one's ability to demonstrate skill in the practice of eloquence: the ability to find the right words to disclose the truth of the matters at hand and to do so in such a way that an audience is moved to better understand and appreciate the revelation that is taking form. Johnson admits that these rhetorical concerns were on her mind when she accepted Singer's invitation: "[I]t seemed an unusual opportunity to experiment with modes of discourse that might work with very tough audiences and bridge the divide between [disability activists'] perceptions and theirs. I didn't expect to straighten out Singer's head, but maybe I could reach a student or two." Moreover, she "was sure [that the experience] would make a great story, first for telling and then for writing down" (1).

Now comes the experience with Singer, which Johnson has been sharing since the beginning of her essay. Remember, this piece of public moral argument is the result of her putting her thoughts together after she returned from Princeton. Johnson tells us that what stands out when she recalls her first meeting with Singer "is his apparent immunity to my looks, his apparent lack of discombobulation, his immediate ability to deal with me as a person with a particular point of view" (2). This first meeting occurred not at Princeton but at a lecture that Singer was giving in South Carolina, at the College of Charleston. Johnson attended the lecture as a reporter for Not Dead Yet. What she continues to tell us about her encounter with Singer provides additional background material for understanding his and her characters. Knowing more about their characters adds to an appreciation of the Princeton experience.

Johnson is introduced to Singer before his lecture begins. She writes: "Singer extends his hand. I hesitate. I shouldn't shake hands with the Evil One. . . .

Hereabouts, the rule is that if you're not prepared to shoot on sight, you have to be prepared to shake hands. I give Singer the three fingers on my right hand that still work. . . . When he says he looks forward to an interesting exchange [after his lecture], he seems entirely sincere" (2). Johnson offers a summary account of the lecture, emphasizing how Singer "spins out his bone-chilling argument" for euthanizing infants who are severely disabled. During the question-and-answer session, Johnson counters the logical and existential inconsistencies of Singer's argument and makes sure he and the audience know "that the presence or absence of a disability doesn't predict quality of life" (3). The exchange between Johnson and Singer goes on for ten minutes. Johnson's description and assessment of their interaction is worth quoting in full.

> He responds to each point with clear and lucid counterarguments. He proceeds with the assumption that I am one of the people who might rightly have been killed at birth. He sticks to his guns, conceding just enough to show himself open-minded and flexible. . . . Even as I am horrified by what he says, and by the fact that I have been sucked into a civil discussion of whether I ought to exist, I can't help being dazzled by his verbal facility. He is so respectful, so free of condescension, so focused on the argument, that by the time the show is over, I'm not exactly angry with him. Yes, I am shaking, furious, enraged—but it's for the big room, 200 of my fellow Charlestonians who have listened with polite interest, when in decency they should have run him out of town on a rail. (3)

Notice that Johnson is taken with Singer's civility. He does everything that the interruption that we are calls us to do: he is open and acknowledging, promotes a communal relationship with Johnson, and is rhetorically competent. He is considerate and forbearing as he listens to what Johnson has to say. He is a good man but somebody who should be run out of town because he is evil. The assessment interrupts itself, encouraging pause for thought: Johnson considers Singer to be rotten with perfection. Singer considers severely disabled infants to be rotten with imperfections since, according to his philosophy of Preference Utilitarianism, they lack the essential features of personhood: "they cannot see themselves as beings that might or might not have a future." They thereby "cannot have a desire to want to go on living." Moreover, "if a right to life must be based on the capacity to want to go on living, or on the ability to see oneself as a continuing mental subject, a newborn baby cannot have the right to life." Finally, "a newborn baby is not an autonomous being, capable of making choices, and so to kill a newborn baby cannot violate the principle of respect for autonomy." And with this reasoning in mind, it makes sense to say that "the newborn baby is on the same footing as the fetus," which also lacks the essential features of personhood.[15] According to Singer, without any degree of personhood we are like snails. "Killing a snail does not thwart any desires of [betterment] because snails are incapable of having such desires."[16] Singer maintains that people with disabilities must be defended, but these people may be so devoid of personhood that it would be better for all concerned to euthanize them. Eventually, this action would eliminate the problem of disability for future generations. In the best of all possible worlds, disability would be nonexistent. Why make disabled people suffer any more than they already have, especially if the suffering is complicated by the patient's rightful belief that his or her suffering is adding to the immense suffering of others? In arguing for the morality of acknowledging and supporting the wishes of people who have a rationally based interest in wanting to end their lives, including parents who would abort a fetus because of its diagnosed disabilities, Singer never advocates that we have an obligation to perform such acts. Relying on our well-reasoned interests and our ability to articulate them in some meaningful way, we must make the choice.

The person saying all of this, to repeat Johnson's comment, is "so respectful, so free of condescension, so focused on the argument" and, as she knows full well, rotten with perfection. Johnson didn't have to share this perception, but it is a rhetorically competent thing to do. The contrast is evocative. Singer is an oxymoron: His goodness is evil.

After the session, Johnson and Singer make arrangements to keep the conversation going over email. Of the many things that are said during the conversation, this statement by Johnson is most striking: "Are we 'worse off'? I don't think so. Not in any meaningful sense. There are too many variables. For those of us with congenital conditions, disability shapes all of us. Those disabled later in life adapt. We take constraints that no one would choose and hold rich and satisfying lives within them. We enjoy pleasures other people enjoy, and pleasures peculiarly our own. We have something that the world needs" (4).

I am taken with the eloquence of this last point. Given all of the background we now have about how she has dealt with the interruption that we are, it should be clear how her story defines a major part of the narrative of her life, how her illness defines significant aspects of her personhood, how her personhood informs and is informed by her narrative, and how this narrative speaks of something that the world needs: a heartfelt appreciation of the value of open-mindedness, acknowledgment, community, and the rhetorical competence to disclose the truth in a moving way. The earlier quoted words of Rabbi Abraham Heschel come to mind: A self "insists not only on being satisfied but also on being able to satisfy, on *being a need* not only on *having needs.* Personal needs come and go, but one anxiety remains: *Am I needed?*" Harriet McBryde Johnson is needed.

Before they decide to end the conversation, Singer invites Johnson to Princeton and she accepts, although she feels rather uneasy because she knows that the disability community "should not legitimate Singer's views by giving them a forum. We should not make disabled lives subject to debate" (4). Johnson shares a few details about the burdens involved for a disabled person who is preparing to board a plane. Having reached her hotel in Princeton, the burdens continue the morning of her presentations as she readies herself—with the help of personal assistant, Carmen—to meet Singer and his students: "I let myself be propped up [in bed] to eat oatmeal and drink tea. Then there's the bedpan and then bathing and dressing, still in bed. Carmen lifts me into my chair and straps a rolled towel under my ribs for comfort and stability. She tugs at my clothes to remove wrinkles that could cause pressure sores" (6). Singer doesn't tell these types of person stories. He doesn't have the requisite experience. If, however, he were disabled like Johnson and still held fast to his philosophy of Preference Utilitarianism, he certainly would have a stronger case. But then, of course, his interests (or, initially, those of others) would have already led to his death. The matter would be moot.

At this point in the story I ask my students whether they like what Johnson has to say so far about her life, its benefits and burdens, her assessment of Singer, and her use of the right words to disclose the truth of these matters of concern. The judgments are never all totally positive, but the majority of the undergraduates, graduates, physicians, lawyers, and health-care associates agree that Johnson tells a "good" story. For example: It's "coherent," "evocative," "disturbing," and "intelligent." Her "biting humor" makes the seriousness of her argument "compelling" and "effective." As one might expect, she knows how to construct a "moving account" of the health of a disabled person's lived body. And her way of using interruption to tell the truth about Singer—he is a good and an evil man—is a creative use of the perfectionist impulse of language. The students agree that Johnson is an interruption who has been exposed to the interruption that we are, is struggling to make the best use of the interruption's perfective impulse, is being interrupted by people influenced by a narrative that grants power to the interruption's defeatist impulse, and who is dedicated to constructing an interruptive counternarrative that informs these people of the error of their ways. I then ask the students whether they would want to be Johnson and whether, if they knew that they were going to give birth to an infant with severe disabilities, they would follow Singer's solution. None of the students want to be Johnson. The majority lean toward Singer's solution. Those who abide by the doctrine of the sanctity of life are the exceptions. My final question before we move on is this: Do you think it is important for Johnson to engage in public moral argument about the topic of disability rights even if the audience is composed of people who, like you, would never want to live like her? "Without a doubt" is the 100 percent reply. The students and I deal more with this question when we finish Johnson's story.

Johnson begins detailing her experience at Princeton as she tells us, "My talk to the students is pretty Southern. I've decided to pound them with heart, hammer them with narrative and say 'y'all' and 'folks.' I play with the emotional tone, giving them little peaks and valleys, modulating three times in one 45-second pitch. I talk about justice, even beauty and love. I figure they haven't been getting much of that from Singer. . . . Of course I give them some argument too. . . . And woven throughout the talk is the presentation of myself as a representative of a minority group that has been rendered invisible by prejudice and oppression, a participant in a discussion that would not occur in a just world" (6).

Johnson continues by offering some brief remarks about the questions that students raised concerning her arguments against selective infanticide. She expands on a particular question on "keeping alive the unconscious." She answers the question by telling a story "about a family . . . which took loving care of a nonresponsive teenage girl, acting out their unconditional commitment to each other, making all the other children, and me as their visitor, feel safe." Singer finds the story insufficient. He responds: "Let's assume we can prove, absolutely, that the individual is totally unconscious and that we can know, absolutely, that the individual will never regain consciousness. Assuming all that, don't you think continuing to take care of that individual would be a bit—weird?'" Johnson responds: "No, done right, it could be profoundly beautiful'" (7).

Elaine Scarry's provocative and insightful assessment of beauty stresses this very point. Something deemed beautiful, argues Scarry, creates "the aspiration for enduring certitude [perfection]." It "calls" for the "perceptual acuity" (acknowledgment) that enables us to appreciate as perfectly as possible some object's or subject's disclosure, its truth, and thereby to appropriate and cultivate the knowledge and wisdom made possible by this revelation. Scarry offers a wonderful example for the teacher and rhetorician.

> [T]here is no way to be in a high state of alert toward injustices—to subjects that, because they entail injuries, will bring distress—without simultaneously demanding of oneself precisely the level of perceptual acuity that will forever be opening one to the arrival of beautiful sights and sounds. How will one even notice, let alone become concerned about, the inclusion in a political assembly of only one economic point of view unless one has also attended, with full acuity, to a debate that is itself a beautiful object, full of arguments, counterarguments, wit, spirit, ripostes, ironies, testing, contesting; and how in turn will one hear the nuances of even this debate unless one also makes oneself available to the songs of birds or poets?[17]

Scarry emphasizes that acknowledgment is attuned to the "aliveness" of a person or object, an aliveness that makes the object's "abrasive handling seem unthinkable. The mind recoils—as from a wound cut into living flesh." The recoil gives us pause for concerned thought. Beauty "incites deliberation." What is brought to mind here "is not the level of aliveness, which is already absolute, but one's own access to the already existing level of aliveness, bringing about, if not a perfect match, at least a less inadequate match between the actual aliveness of others and the level with which we daily credit them." Scarry thus maintains that beauty places "requirements on us for attending to the aliveness . . . of our world, and for entering into its protection."[18] Meeting these requirements helps to establish the "justice" that is needed if we intend to treat other people and other things with heartfelt concern and respect.

Johnson has nothing more to say about her first presentation. Rather, she talks about her "walk around campus" with Singer before she gives her second presentation. When discussing her topic during that presentation, Johnson admits that "What worries me most about the proposal for legalized assisted suicide is its veneer of beneficence—the medical determination that, for a given individual, suicide is reasonable or right. It is not about autonomy but about nondisabled people telling us what's good for us" (8). Johnson gives no indication in this or any other response she offers during the presentation of anger and frustration. On the contrary, she credits herself as having been particularly civil to the company she kept while at Princeton. When she returns home and shares her experience with friends, "they worry that my civility may have given Singer a new kind of legitimacy." She asks herself a "tough question": "am I in fact a silly little lady whose head is easily turned by a man who gives her a kind of attention she enjoys? I hope not, but I confess that I've never been able to sustain righteous anger for more than about 30 minutes at a time. My view of life tends more toward tragedy" (9). She admits, however, that Singer "is a man of unusual gifts, reaching for the heights. He writes that he is trying to create a system of ethics derived from fact and reason, that largely throws off the perspectives of religion, place, family, tribe, community and maybe even species—to 'take the point of view of the universe.' His is a grand, heroic undertaking," despite his "flaw" of believing "that disabled people are inherently 'worse off,' that we 'suffer,' that we have lesser 'prospects of a happy life.'" Still, "I can't look at him without fellow-feeling" (9).

More than ever, Johnson is responding to the call of the interruption that we are. She is open to Singer, acknowledging his presence, establishing a communal bond with him, and displaying rhetorical competence in the polite way she is conversing with him and his students. Yet the fact remains. Johnson is a disability activist whose life would have ended in the womb if Singer had his say. This is the point that her associates stress: "Singer doesn't deserve my human sympathy. I should make him an object of implacable wrath, to be cut off, silenced, destroyed absolutely. And I find myself lacking a logical argument to the contrary" (9–10).

According to the journalist Johann Hari, who interviewed Singer in 2004, the man "is not a drooling, swastika-waving eugenicist, whatever his foes say."[19] So why, he asks, do they hate him? Hari quotes Singer's answer to the question: "We are living in an incredible time of transition. In the West, we have been dominated by a single tradition for 2,000 years. Now that whole tradition, the whole edifice of Judeo-Christian morality, is terminally ill. I am trying to formulate an alternative. Some of what I say seems obscene and evil if you are still looking at it through the prism of the old morality. That's what happens when morality shifts: people get confused and angry and disgusted." Hari's reaction to the reasoning displayed in Singer's rhetoric is noteworthy: "Singer is pure, disembodied rationality—the Enlightenment made flesh. He measures pain and capacity to suffer in neat units and disregards old-fangled notions such as species or emotion. He discusses killing babies . . . with the passion of a speaking-clock." Hari ends the interview with a remark with which I identify: "Give me Singer over the Vatican-style superstitions he is trying to dispel any day; and yet, as I leave the interview, I can't shake off a strange—Singer would say sentimental—anxiety."[20]

Johnson concludes her story as she tells of a phone conversation with her sister Beth, who was incensed with Singer and his reasoning and rhetoric. Johnson attempts to show some understanding for her opponent's position. Beauty and justice are evident—as is hope. Despite his honest commitment to his cause, Singer uses rhetoric that, writes Johnson, "won't matter in the end. He won't succeed in reinventing morality. He stirs the pot, brings things out into the open. But ultimately we'll make a world that's fit to live in, a society that has room for all its flawed creatures. History will remember Singer as a curious example of the bizarre things that can happen when paradigms collide" (10). Beth's criticism is not receptive to such a hopeful outlook. "What if you wind up in a world where the disabled person's 'irrational' preference to live must yield to society's 'rational' interest in reducing the incidence of disability? Doesn't horror kick in somewhere? Maybe as you watch the door close behind whoever has wheeled you into the gas chamber?" (10). Johnson responds with an instructive, eloquent, and moving insight filled with heartfelt honesty and sincerity:

> If I define Singer's kind of disability prejudice as an ultimate evil, and him as a monster, then I must so define all who believe disabled lives are inherently worse off or that a life without a certain kind of consciousness lacks value. That definition would make monsters of many of the people with whom I move on the sidewalks, do business, break bread, swap stories and share the grunt work of local politics. It would reach some of my family and most of my nondisabled friends, people who show me personal kindness and who sometimes manage to love me through their ignorance. I can't

> live with a definition of ultimate evil that encompasses all of them. I can't refuse the monster-majority basic respect and human sympathy. It's not in my heart to deny every single one of them, categorically, my affection and my Love. . . . My fight has been for accommodation, the world to me and me to the world. As a disability pariah, I must struggle for a place for kinship, for community, for connection. . . . My goal isn't to shed the perspective that comes from my particular experience, but to give voice to it. I want to be engaged in the tribal fury that rages when opposing perspectives are let loose. . . . I'll invoke the muck and mess and undeniable reality of disabled lives well lived. That's the best I can do. (11)

Disability activists live lives that are incomprehensible to far too many nondisabled people. These activists, committed to disclosing the truth of who they are, need to find the right words that can help people comprehend the incomprehensible and make unspeakable conversations speakable. The right words can open up people to others. The right words can foster acknowledgment and communal relationships. The right words display the rhetorical competence that is called for by the interruption that we are. The answer to an earlier question is obvious. One cannot stress enough the importance of disability rights activists engaging in public moral argument about the health of their lived bodies, even if their audience would never change places with these activists. The right words might at least help remedy a problem noted by Johnson in her story: "most people don't know how to look at me." The perfective impulse of the interruption that we are must be put to use if its defeatist impulse is not to have its way. Controlled by this impulse, people give up on life and any joys it has to offer. They even are known to say, "I wish I were dead." Disability activists eliminated this phrase from their narrative of the good life. Johnson's story gives voice to this narrative.

When Johnson died, the *New York Times* invited Singer to write an obituary, which he did. Not Dead Yet was outraged. The disability activist Paul Longmore wrote: "[W]e who mourn the loss of our Harriet must regard this obituary as not just falsifying but obscene."[21] I find nothing false about the obituary. Given its author, however, the piece certainly can be obscene to members of the disability community. I have a different reading of the obituary. It is ten paragraphs long, the first nine detailing the history of Johnson's relationship with Singer. Nothing wrong or strange there. On the contrary, Singer recalls reading Johnson's "Unspeakable Conversations" and her trip to Princeton, and he shares these thoughts: "She wrote beautifully, her powers of recollection were remarkable (she wasn't taking notes at the time) and she was more generous to me than I had a right to expect from someone whose very existence I had questioned. She even wrote that she found me good company, as indeed I found her."[22] The compliment interrupts an otherwise nonemotional account, until the last paragraph, where another, more evocative interruption occurs. The words that define this interruption are not those of a speaking clock. Singer writes: "According to her sister, Beth, what most concerned Harriet about dying was 'the crap people would say about her.' And, sure enough, among the tributes to her were several comments about how she can now run and skip through the meadows of heaven. Doubly insulting, first because Johnson did not believe in a life after death, and second, why assume that heavenly bliss requires you to be able to run and skip?"

These final words, and especially the last sentence, are, at least for me, evidence that Johnson found some right words to affect in a positive way a non-compromising opponent of her stance on eugenics and euthanasia. In order for Singer to conclude his obituary as he does, he had to have been moved to be open to, acknowledge, and form some communal ties with Johnson. Her rhetorical competence also was successful enough to help Singer *know how to look* at Johnson so that he could accurately appreciate what she considered to be the health of her lived body and how it should not be demeaned by ill-conditioned and wrongheaded thinking. Indeed, Johnson didn't consider being able to run and skip as credible criteria for gauging the intelligence, lively emotional disposition, and dignity of her personhood. Singer had a heart for Johnson. The perfective impulse of the interruption that we are was put to good use by one self saying farewell to another self who had dedicated her life to using this impulse in a most praiseworthy way. The self as other. The other as self. Public moral argument provided an opportunity for this transformation to occur.

CHAPTER 6

A Good Showing of a Bad Situation

> "Choices about death touch the core of liberty. Our duty, and the concomitant freedom to come to terms with the conditions of our own mortality are undoubtedly 'so rooted in the traditions and conscience of our people as to be ranked as fundamental' . . . and indeed are essential incidents of the unalienable right to life and liberty endowed by our Creator."
>
> John Paul Stevens, *Cruzan v. Director, Missouri Department of Health*

....

Harriet McBryde Johnson wanted people to see, think, and acknowledge her as a normal person who, perhaps like them, enjoyed being alive. She was determined to achieve those goals for herself and fellow disability activists, who regarded her as a "hero."[1] My students agree with this evaluation but still would not want to live her life. Recalling a statement made to Johnson by a passerby—"If I had to live like you, I think I'd kill myself"—I ask the students if they feel the same way. We are now talking about suicide, a term that has such negative connotations and interruptive force that it provokes extended pause for thought. Some students find this option acceptable, others are quite hesitant. I pose another scenario. You have an incurable disease that is causing tortuous pain and mental distress. Medications offer some relief but not enough. Your life is void of any quality, and you learn that the progressive nature of the disease gives you at most six more months to live. You are more than ever before exposed to the interruption that we are. The majority of students are now more open to the option of suicide, but they admit that it would be "a lonely and bad way to go," not a "good death." We have a term for this depiction: euthanasia, from the Greek *eu* (good) *thanatos* (death), which is typically associated with a physician heeding the request of a suffering patient and using drugs to assist the patient die a painless death. The practice is termed "active euthanasia" or "physician-assisted suicide." Other terms include "voluntary euthanasia," "death with dignity," "physician aid in dying," and "medical aid in dying." Four states (Oregon, Washington, Vermont, and California) have legalized this practice, and the rules governing the practice are strict and extensive.[2]

The social acceptability and justifiability of euthanasia continue to be among the most controversial issues in medical ethics and bioethics. The following example shows why. In the summer of 2016, I was involved in a field research project that included the case of an eighty-five-year-old woman (call her Fran) dying of bone cancer and who consented to be housed in a hospice facility. Four days before she died, she requested a consultation with her physician, who had treated her for the past year and whom she trusted more than any other of her physicians. This physician was exceptionally kind and caring, especially when it came to listening to all that Fran had to say. During their conversation, Fran admitted that she was afraid to die because, being a devout Christian, she felt that she had yet to become worthy of being accepted into heaven. She needed more time to stay alive and wanted to restart her chemotherapy. Her physician explained to her that being a hospice patient prevented any more invasive treatment and, besides, more chemo would further endanger her life. Her response was a major interruption: "But without the chemo, aren't I committing suicide?"

The physician made clear that suicide was an improper way to think about her situation, that she should not worry because she was a good Christian, and that the rest of her days would be peaceful. The staff began treating her with morphine every four hours and then at two-hour intervals. Fran died two days later. It was a good death, with Fran having received assistance all along from her physician, the hospice nurses and staff, her chaplain, and her four children, who took turns staying with her overnight during the last two weeks so that she felt secure. They all *assisted* her in dying a good death. Hence, they all engaged in the practice of passive euthanasia. This practice is confined to the withholding or withdrawing of life-sustaining technologies; death is brought about by the underlying disease. Hospice physicians and medical staff take great exception to being associated with any form of euthanasia, given the ongoing debate over its ethical status and the negative connotations of the term. From my point of view, however, passive euthanasia defines the ultimate goal of hospice care.

Singer is an advocate of voluntary euthanasia. So, for example, he maintains that "the principle of respect for autonomy tells us to allow rational agents to live their own lives according to their own autonomous decisions, free from coercion or interference; but if rational agents should autonomously choose to die, then respect for autonomy will lead us to assist them to do as they choose."[3] Johnson takes exception to the practice because it can add to the problem of "disability discrimination," whereby society provides a way to rid itself of disabled people who have yet to find the proper assistance to live a good life and thus find euthanasia the only remedy for the deteriorating health of their lived bodies.[4] Johnson's assessment of the ethics of euthanasia is always offered in the context of disability rights. That's her choice, and it warrants respect. Singer would certainly agree. Yet, in privileging that choice, the rhetoric of the right-to-die movement, which I mentioned earlier, is discredited as being but a danger to the disability community. In all fairness, however, this rhetoric and the narrative it sustains are also about disabled individuals whose lived bodies are devastated by disease and the pain and suffering that go with the disease. Their lives have become a living death. Euthanasia advocates make much of how such an existential state is more often than not a "horror" story for patients and their loved ones. If a patient wants to end this story because it "only is going to get worse" for all concerned, why not help her conclude the final chapter with whatever human dignity she has left? The bioethicist Ronald Green offers an instructive answer to this question.

Green points out that one's decision to die, the choice to "cease being a choosing being," is not patently absurd or irrational. "Life involves many choices that have the effect of foreclosing future choices of the same kind, and the choice of death or a course leading to death is only the most extreme of these. . . . We must not forget," Green argues, "that for some persons 'dignity' does have the meaning of not spending their last days being treated like an infant or a noisome inanimate object, or of not being subjected to conditions that disempower them and alter their personality so as to render them unrecognizable to their loved ones."[5] Dying with dignity does not merely put an end to dignity; it also may demonstrate and serve as a reminder of its own essential worth. Being the ultimate sacrifice, dying with dignity can define a holy act (*sacer facere*, 'to make holy')—one that allows a patient (before it is too late) a last chance to take some control over the final chapter of her life. Life and death are inextricably related. If one has been fortunate enough to have lived something of the good life, then dying a good death allows goodness to continue up to the very end. Moreover, such an ending pays homage to the good life of others and their need for stories that, as much as possible, have a good ending. Dying with dignity is a demonstration of a person's moral integrity. The philosopher Martin Foss puts the matter well: "Sacrifice, even if it is a sacrificial death, is not an end but a transition to a new beginning. It is an offering which in its passing way is somehow preserved because it integrates and intensifies that for which it was an offering. In the sacrificial deed, that which is seemingly destroyed is made to live on and is thus not only preserved, but—more than that—it is elevated [*dignitas*] and plays a role in a higher sphere of meaning. Here is destruction which turns into creation; it is an end which converts into a beginning and has meaning beyond mere destruction."[6] In short, the choice to die with dignity warrants being seen as a heroic act.

The philosopher and bioethicist Leon Kass rejects the arguments of those like Green and Foss. He notes: "One can *sympathize* with [a person's request for euthanasia] out of compassion, but can one admire it, out of respect? Is it really dignified to seek to escape from troubles for oneself? Is there . . . not more dignity in courage than in its absence? . . . How can I honor myself by making myself nothing?"[7] But is the issue here simply that of honoring oneself? What about others? Kass addresses this last question with a series of additional questions: "Is it dignified to ask or demand that someone else become my killer? It may be said that one is unable to end one's own life, but can it conduce to either party's dignity to make the request? Consider its double meaning if made to a son or daughter: Do you love me so little as to force me to live on? Do you love me so little as to want me dead? What person in full possession of his or her own dignity would inflict such a duty on anyone they loved?"[8]

With this last question in mind, advocates of the right to die point to a self whose relationship with loved ones is informed by a shared knowledge that values the acknowledgment and love that come with the sacrifice of being for others. It is a matter of having a heart for a self who has a heart for others.[9] The dignity and moral integrity of a self can benefit and instruct others so that they, in turn, become more dependable and competent selves when responding to the call of others. The matter at hand brings Levinas to mind. The person opting for euthanasia is a self in desperate need of help. This self is thus an other whose exposure to the interruption that we are incites a call of conscience. For Levinas, we have an ethical obligation not to remain indifferent to this call, "not to let the other die alone," but instead "to answer for the life of the other person, at the risk of becoming an accomplice in that person's death."[10] The self is obliged to respond to the other, who at any moment can become a self faced with the same obligation.

The related issues of dignity and moral integrity lie at the heart of the euthanasia debate. Those aligned with the right-to-life movement use the term "physician-assisted suicide" when engaged in public moral argument about the justifiability of seeking the good death. The negative connotation of suicide works to their favor. Those aligned with the right-to-die movement use various other terms—"physician aid in dying," "death with dignity," "medical aid in dying"—that reflect what they maintain is a more truthful interpretation of the matter than what their opponents would have us believe. In the euthanasia debate, it is crucial for each side to have people think that they have the right words for accurately assessing the health of the lived body. The perfectionist impulse of language warrants serious consideration. Rhetorical competence is expected.

The case that concerns us now—the story of Brittany Maynard—offers a vivid illustration of the performance of this task. In January 2014, Maynard was exposed to the interruption that we are. She was diagnosed with terminal brain cancer, which led to an eight-hour brain surgery. In April she was told by physicians that she had six months to live. She was twenty-nine years old. She was a medical-aid-in-dying advocate.[11] She and her husband moved from California to Oregon, where medical aid in dying is legal. In accordance with Oregon's "Death with Dignity" law, she requested and received from a physician a lethal prescription of medicine that she could ingest to end her dying process if it became unbearable. Before the full force of her cancer materialized, she took the medication while lying in bed. Her husband, mother, and other loved ones were there to comfort her as she passed away, on November 1, 2014.

Drawing on friendships she made while attending a wedding in California in July 2014, Maynard agreed to have them make a short video of her talking about her situation. The video included earlier pictures of Maynard and brief remarks from her husband and mother. Her account is the rhetorical construction of a narrative that details her progression from a vibrant life to one of cancer-ridden suffering, makes clear how she plans to deal with the disease, and emphasizes the need to expand medical-aid-in-dying laws nationwide. Maynard is a wounded storyteller whose exposure to the interruption that we are led her to favor the interruption's perfective impulse. It was an act of authenticity, of self-determination. Her video placed her dignity and moral integrity on the line. Judgment was forthcoming.

When Maynard and her husband returned to Oregon, the video was eventually shared with the end-of-life organization Compassion & Choices. On October 6, 2014, by way of People.com, Maynard partnered with this organization and released the six-and-a-half-minute video.[12] The video went viral, and Maynard's story was credited with putting a "new face" on the medical-aid-in-dying movement. Barbara Coombs Lee, coauthor of Oregon's medical-aid-in-dying law and president of Compassion & Choices, justifies this characterization of the video when she notes: "The general public has sort of an unspoken expectation that [medical aid in dying] is what old people deal with. Brittany Maynard's situation is so much different. She's young; she's vibrant. She could be my daughter. She could be a granddaughter, a neighbor, a school friend."[13] To understand fully all that this situation entails, one must attend not only to Maynard's youth but also, and more important, to how she tells her story about her life and upcoming death. The development of the story is public moral argument in the making.

More than 400,000 people visited People.com to view Maynard's video on the first day it was available. Maynard and various supporters of her cause appeared in additional videos and interviews to speak about and clarify her situation and to argue for the legality of medical aid in dying. She became a nationally and internationally known figure. Her story, from beginning to end, was considered heroic.[14] In the much-publicized cases of Nancy Cruzan (1983–1990) and Terri Schiavo (1990–2005), family members and doctors communicated on behalf of the patients. Medical circumstances prevented the patients from participating in the dialogue regarding their health and wishes. Brittany Maynard's situation was different. Public moral argument became an activity in self-advocacy.

Maynard's story is an ethical and rhetorical endeavor to make a good showing of a bad situation, which, as performed by a wounded storyteller, entails a commitment of living for others. Recall Arthur Frank's directive that a wounded storyteller constructs a narrative meant to benefit herself and others in need of education about the health of their lived bodies. The way in which Maynard's story takes form and develops is unprecedented in the historical debate over the (im)morality of euthanasia.[15] Those who take issue with the story seek to make sure that the new face of the medical-aid-in-dying movement is not without blemishes. Worlds of know-how are conflicting with each other.

Brittany Maynard

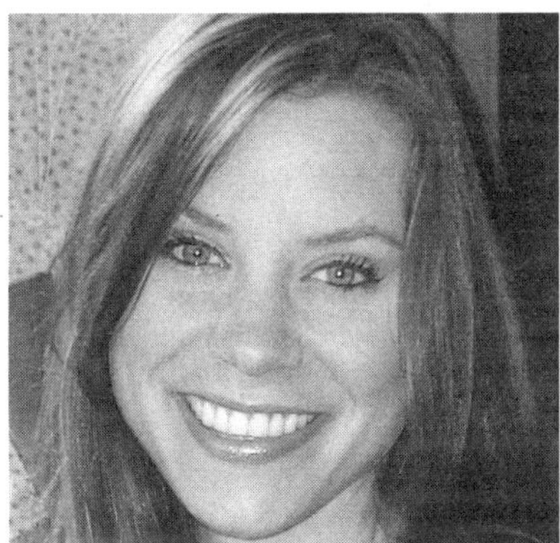

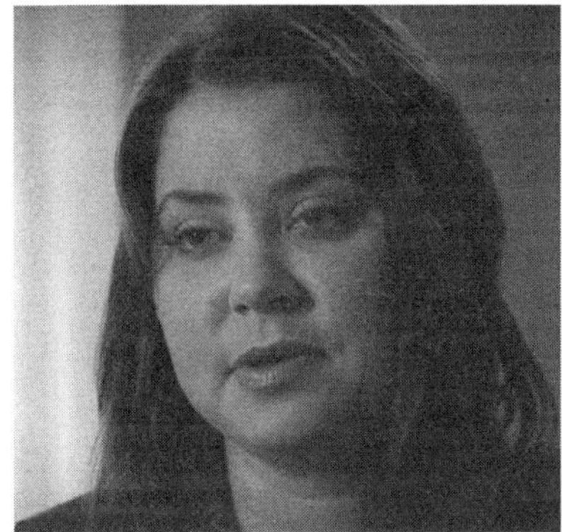

The face on the left is Maynard when her cancer had yet to ravage her brain. The face on the right is Maynard suffering the consequences of medication designed to reduce inflammation in her brain. She had gained more than twenty-five pounds as the result of her medications The physical appearance of the faces is incongruent. Owing to this incongruence one is likely not to know, when seeing them for the first time, that they belong to the same person. Maynard's first video corrects this impression as it begins disclosing her current predicament with brain cancer, how this predicament relates to her recent past, and how she intends to deal with her illness. As discussed later, the correction makes the incongruence rhetorically significant, thereby helping a wounded storyteller involve herself in the ethical activity of communicating with others who can benefit from what she has to say.

The video opens with a shot of Maynard's face, after her diagnosis of brain cancer. This is the face we see most often as Maynard begins and continues her story. The next brief set of frames contains words on black screens. "In January

2014, after years of suffering from debilitating headaches, Brittany Maynard found out that she had brain cancer. . . . She was given a prognosis of six months left to live. She had recently turned 29." Several frames of Maynard's marriage ceremony and celebration then appear, exposing for the first time in the video her physical appearance before it was changed by her cancer treatments. The exposure is striking. The face presented in the marriage scenes is incongruent with the face that has been speaking so far. The conflict heightens our consciousness of a tragic situation. R. Buckminster Fuller is correct: The workings of consciousness are incited by an "awareness of otherness. . . . And all statements by consciousness are in the comparative terms of prior observations of consciousness ('It's warmer, it's quicker, it's bigger than others'). . . . Consciousness dawns with the second experience."[16] The incongruent faces in the video produce this experience, which played a key role in Maynard's reception by the public. Critics declared that she did not look that sick in the video. Dan Diaz, Maynard's widower, addressed these critics by explaining that although she appeared healthy, her health was constantly deteriorating, with seizures taking away her ability to communicate for hours at a time.[17]

Maynard does not comment on how her looks have changed because of her cancer treatments. Given its effect on the viewer's consciousness, the change is, however, rhetorically significant. To repeat an earlier quoted insight of Henry Johnstone: "*Rhetoric is the evocation and the maintenance of the consciousness required for communication.*"[18] To the extent that it successfully performs this function, rhetoric deserves credit for producing a good showing of its subject matter, one that is interesting, thought-provoking, and enlightening; encourages wise judgment; and is persuasive with all that it has to say about its subject—hence the effectiveness of rhetoric.

The effectiveness of the Maynard video's presentation of the changes to her physical appearance facilitates the production of what Kenneth Burke terms a "perspective by incongruity." The power of this rhetorical maneuver is demonstrated as it serves to heighten one's consciousness of the video's central concern: the story of Brittany Maynard.[19] The maneuver speaks to us of an exceptionally sad situation: the inevitable death of a young woman dying from a horrific disease. The sadness increases as Maynard tells us that "Right when I was diagnosed my husband and I were actively trying for a family which is heartbreaking for us both." A wounded storyteller's tragic situation is vividly apparent.

The remainder of Maynard's first video furthers the feeling of sadness associated with her illness and its consequences. For example, we see Maynard removing from her purse the pills that will help bring about her death. We hear from Maynard how her mother was hoping for a "miracle." Maynard describes the scene she envisions when she dies in her bed. The last words we hear on the video are those of Maynard, having less than a month to live: "I hope to enjoy how many days I have on this earth and spend as much of it outside as I can, surrounded by those I love. The reason to consider life and what's of value is to make sure that you are not missing out. Seize the day, what's important to you, what do you care about, what matters. Pursue that. Forget the rest." This is spirited advice, but it also serves as a reminder that a young woman's wisdom is ending too soon. Sadness prevails, facilitated early on by a rhetorical maneuver that functions to heighten one's consciousness of the plight of a wounded storyteller. The new face of the medical-aid-in-dying movement is being constructed. Indeed, a perspective by incongruity lends itself to making a good showing of a bad situation.

In a video released two days before she died, Maynard addresses an issue that is not mentioned in her first video or, as far as I know, in any other of her videos. I refer to her physical presence. As in her first video, the second video shows Maynard telling her story while various pictures appear showing her wedding ceremony and other joyful moments in her life. The incongruence of her physical appearance is obvious. She admits as much: "It's a weird feeling to wake up every day and be in my body because it feels so different than it did just a year ago. . . . I don't like being photographed, I don't like being filmed, and I don't like spending a lot of time looking in the mirror. And I am not full of self-hate or loathing, it is just that my body has changed so quickly."[20] I think it is fair to say that, despite her dislike of being photographed or filmed and of seeing herself in a mirror, Maynard's remarks are not those of an egotistical and vain individual. She is bothered by her looks but not enough to refuse to be filmed for a cause that she sees as having undeniable worth. Her growing emotional distress is associated first and foremost with her sickness and its death sentence.

Anatole Broyard wrote about the communicative activity of a wounded storyteller as he was dying from metastatic cancer. He emphasizes that "To remain silent is literally to close down the ship of one's humanity."[21] The storyteller's ability to make a good showing of her subject matter requires the teller to engage in the inventive process of finding a way with words that make an audience more receptive to the teller's teachings. It is the ethical thing to do and, to be sure, the rhetorical thing to do. Eloquence is required. Kenneth Burke identifies an essential feature of this phenomenon when noting that the eloquent speaker "seeks to make sure that his observations, arguments, and overall prose are firmly grounded in the situation at hand." Burke thus emphasizes, as quoted earlier, that "The primary purpose of eloquence is to 'convert life' to its most thorough verbal equivalent."[22] Seen this way, eloquence has a role to play in establishing a person's moral integrity.

Maynard employs what is known as the "plain style" of eloquence.[23] This style consists of prose that is simple, direct, and unambiguous. The eloquence of the plain style, its way with words, is "straight talk" that abides by the approved social attributes favored by an audience listening to a wounded storyteller talking about her unrecoverable illness and its consequences. Plain-style eloquence is a fitting and thus appropriate response to such a heartbreaking situation in that it avoids language that draws attention toward its own ornate nature and away from the somber and urgent matter at hand: the sadness generated by the perspective by incongruity in Maynard's first video and that continues to play a role throughout her story. "The gift of proper expression [eloquence]," writes Georges Gusdorf, "is the privilege of certain beings who intuitively know the balance-point and show, in the face of the most unexpected difficulty, that they are equal to the circumstances."[24] Moreover, plain-style eloquence facilitates an audience's belief in the rhetor's sincerity, which helps to validate the authenticity of the sadness that permeates all that Maynard has to say about her situation.[25]

Sincerity is an admirable quality. It warrants respect. It promotes the perception that the rhetor's discourse is free from pretense and deceit. It enhances the possibility that people will have a heart for the speaker's situation. Adhering to the approved social attributes favored by an audience, a rhetor's employment of the plain style risks what Burke maintains is the temptation to rely solely on language that is familiar and revered.[26] The risk is worth it, however, when a rhetor's sincerity is on the line. Without sincerity, the rhetorical structure of Maynard's story lacks moral integrity, which aids in the construction of a convincing argument for approving the new face of the medical-aid-in-dying movement.[27] Sincerity is needed to make a good showing of a bad situation. Sincerity, of course, can be demonstrated in the discourse of people whose hearts are devoted to evil ends. A person who advocates bone-chilling racist views is a case in point. Sincerity can also be faked.[28]

None of what I reviewed of Maynard telling her story lacks what I consider genuine sincerity. She does not express bias toward anyone. In a commentary for the CNN organization, Maynard offers what I take to be a noteworthy display of plain-style eloquence and its production of sincerity.

> I considered passing away in hospice care. . . . But even with palliative medication, I could develop potentially morphine-resistant pain and suffer personality changes and verbal, cognitive and motor loss of virtually any kind. Because the rest of my body is young and healthy, I am likely to physically hang on for a long time even though cancer is eating my mind. . . . I have had the medication [to end my life] for weeks. I am not suicidal. If I were, I would have consumed that medication long ago. I do not want to die. But I am dying. And I want to die on my own terms. I would not tell anyone else that he or she should choose death with dignity. My question is: Who has the right to tell me that I don't deserve this choice? That I deserve to suffer for weeks or months in tremendous amounts of physical and emotional

> pain. . . . Now that I've had the prescription filled and it's in my possession, I have experienced a tremendous sense of relief. . . . I know that I have a safety net. . . . I hope for the sake of my fellow American citizens that I'll never meet that this option is available to you.[29]

A wounded storyteller is telling it like it is. Her way with words makes clear her humanity, character, and moral integrity. Burke's aforementioned instruction about the function of eloquence is applicable here: Maynard's "observations, arguments, and overall prose are firmly grounded in the situation at hand." Notice, too, that Maynard adheres to Burke's final instruction about eloquence: its "primary purpose . . . is to 'convert life' to its most thorough verbal equivalent." Maynard takes exception to those who equate her decision to die with the disparaging and noxious term "suicide." The term is unfitting given her circumstances. "Death with dignity," not suicide, is the most thorough verbal equivalent of Maynard's situation.[30]

If this use of dignity more eloquently captures the meaning of Maynard's actions, what is dignity? The true meaning of dignity is a major point of contention between Maynard's supporters and critics, for dignity is a quality essential to humankind's well-being and spiritual welfare. Definitions are created by using symbols "to draw a line around" (*definire*) something to mark its meaningful borders. Hence, to define a given term is to set forth a proposal or argument for what the term means. Definitions, in other words, are symbolic (rhetorical) constructions whose most honorable purpose is to make the best use of the perfectionist impulse of language so as to direct people toward the truth.[31] Users of the term "dignity," however, need not define it because just mentioning the term in one's discourse is a dignified thing to do. In and of itself, dignity has rhetorical power, unless recipients of a person's argument take exception to this particular use of power when someone is advocating a position on a controversial issue. Whether they define it or not, people want to have dignity on their side. Like sincerity, dignity warrants respect. People tend to be more mindful of what a dignified person has to say.[32]

Favorable responses to Maynard's position are vast in number. For example, Dr. Marcia Angell, senior lecturer in social medicine at Harvard Medical School and a former editor in chief of the *New England Journal of Medicine,* offers this insight and praise when discounting the characterization of Maynard being suicidal: "We give patients the right to hasten their deaths by refusing dialysis, mechanical ventilation, antibiotics or any other life-sustaining treatment. Why deny them what is essentially the same choice [of death with dignity], especially since it is limited to terminally ill patients? . . . Maynard's death is tragic, but in making her story public with such grace, she has greatly helped future patients who want the same choice."[33] Angell speaks from experience. Her husband, a physician, died from metastatic cancer, knew full well that the pain and suffering would be unbearable, but was denied his request to make use of the option championed by the death-with-dignity movement. Angell is aiding early on in the rhetorical construction of the new face of this movement. She is helping make a good showing of a bad situation. She is living *for* the other.

All that I have been saying so far about the story of Brittany Maynard does not go unchallenged. For example, the Vatican promoted a position that is quite different from Angell's. Monsignor Ignacio Carrasco de Paula calls Maynard's assisted suicide "an absurdity": "This woman [took her own life] thinking she would die with dignity, but this is the error. Suicide is not a good thing. It is a bad thing because it is saying no to life and to everything it means with respect to our mission in the world and toward those around us."[34] Maynard's moral integrity is being called into question.

Notice that both Angell and the Monsignor employ the term "dignity" to advance their opposing arguments without defining the term. The dignified responses to Maynard's actions offered by Angell and the Monsignor inform the public moral argument that emerged as soon as Maynard's first video became viral. Such argument produced undignified responses to Maynard's story from both critics and supporters.

The next series of responses comes from various Internet comment sections. These responses represent the extremity of vitriolic reactions to Maynard's story and set the public debate apart from past cases. The anonymity of Internet comments sections allows people to express their opinions differently from the way they might do so in spaces where their identities are more transparent. This serves as evidence of what moral dialogue on medical aid in dying becomes during the Internet era. For example, after learning the details of Maynard's case, atube4view, a critic of the wounded storyteller, offers this advice: "Exactly what all niggers and wetbacks need to do!" A fitting response to this undignified comment is then offered by Farley Boy: "And anyone with the screen name atube-4view."[35] An example of undignified rhetoric from a Maynard supporter, JohnMWhite ComradeAnon, is this: "God chose for [Maynard] to die a horrible, lingering, miserable death that would cause pain and suffering for her and everyone around her. Screw that guy." And prairiedog JohnMWhite follows up with this comment: "And God gave that scumbag Cheney a second shot at life. . . . I do believe God is dead."[36] With smiles on their faces, bigots, atheists, and those who loath Dick Cheney may find these comments amusing. Besides uncovering the meanness at work in responses to Maynard's story, such comments do nothing constructive to advance public moral argument regarding her decision. On the contrary, they contaminate the rational character that such argument should display. But they can also spur public moral argument intended to rectify the problem.

A more robust and rational critical response to Maynard's "assisted suicide" is offered by William Peace, a member of the board for Not Dead Yet.[37] Focusing on Maynard's first video and incorrectly assuming, as did all of the media coverage of Maynard's story, that the video was made by Compassion & Choices, Peace is particularly irked by what he considers to be the manipulative tactics of this right-to-die organization, which he sees as creating "the slick packaging of [Maynard's] life into a tear jerker like framework. . . . The emotional manipulation via imagery involved is over the top. It is a dodge, a shell game. Replace fact with emotion. Maynard's role is to incite sympathy without thought. . . . The fact she has not added anything new to the debate for or against assisted suicide does not matter." Peace's assault on Maynard's moral integrity is obvious: She let herself be used by Compassion & Choices.[38] The assault continues as Peace ends his article by noting that "There are many paths our lives can take and I for one find it sad Maynard has knowingly allowed herself to become the face of the so-called right to die. I would rather be known for how I live, not the way I died."

I find Peace to be overly critical. What he fails to realize is that the particular presentation of Maynard's story performs a rhetorical function that is productive for debate: evocation. Raphael Demos offers a perceptive description of the phenomenon: "Evocation is the process by which vividness is conveyed; it is the presentation of a viewpoint in such a manner that it becomes real for the public. It is said that argument is a way by which an individual experience is made common property; in fact, an argument has much less persuasive force than the vivid evocation of an experience. The enumeration of all the relevant points in favor of a theory and against its opposite can never be completed; far more effective is it to state a viewpoint in all its concreteness and in all its significant implication, and then stop; the arguments become relevant only after this state has been concluded."[39]

The sadness incited by Maynard's story does not replace fact with emotion. The sadness *is* fact. This emotion is not staged to incite sympathy without thought. It *evokes* thought. Peace's response to Maynard's video proves the point. And claiming that the video does not add anything new to the debate for or against assisted suicide is rather odd. Maynard introduces the issue of youth in the debate. And this issue, given the extent of its public exposure, which is still growing with the influence of Maynard's story, is unprecedented in stimulating public moral argument about a certain way of dying.[40] Abiding by Peace's take on the inauthenticity of the story, one would likely dismiss as mere manipulation the following remarks by Maynard recorded three weeks before and released two days before she died. The remarks are part of a story that is the face of the right to die: "Well if all of my dreams come true, I would somehow survive this. . . . So beyond that, having been an only child for my mother, I want her to recover from this and not break down, you know suffer from any kind of depression.

And my husband is such a lovely man, I want him to, you know, that everyone needs to grieve, but I want him to be happy. So I want him to have a family and I know that that might sound weird, but there is no part of me that wants him to live out the rest of his life with just missing his wife. So I hope he moves on and becomes a father."[41]

I am taken with the eloquence of these remarks. They strike and arouse the heart. Maynard's story warrants more credit than Peace gives it. In comments she sent to the *Diane Rehm Show* on National Public Radio, Maynard noted she was disturbed by claims that "Compassion & Choices had somehow taken advantage of me through 'exploitation' and that I feel compelled to die now based on public expectations. I DO NOT, this is MY choice, I am not that weak. I have the right to change my mind at any time, it is my right." She then emphasizes that the "claim of exploitation is utterly false considering I had gone through the entire process of moving, physician approval for DWD [death with dignity], and filled my prescription before I ever even spoke to anyone at Compassion & Choices about volunteering and decided to share my story."[42] I do side with Peace, however, when he declares: "I rail against a society that applauds people like Maynard who want to die and at the same time undermine the ability of those that need social supports to live a good life."[43] Nothing that Maynard says, however, denies the presence of this problem or favors its continuation.

The academic critic Ashton Ellis sides with Peace in his critique of Maynard's story: "Gone are any considerations about the impact legalizing assisted suicide would have on vulnerable populations such as the poor and the disabled. Not a word is mentioned of how normalizing assisted suicide would alter personal, familial, and professional expectations about when someone should choose death. The issue is boiled down to this: I'm dying of cancer. I want to die now." Ellis recommends a remedy to the problem: "What's needed as we deliberate about assisted suicide is not a razor-thin focus on the exceptionally rare case of a beautiful young woman diagnosed with a particularly aggressive type of cancer. Instead, we need a full and robust discussion about whether it is possible, in principle, to stop one person's *right* to die from becoming another's *duty* to die."[44] Ellis is right to identify omissions in Maynard's story regarding possible consequences of its desired goal of legalizing physician-assisted suicide in all fifty states. Like Peace, he is not content to accept the new face of the medical-aid-in-dying movement. He is not satisfied with this movement's effort to make a good showing of a bad situation. He believes that "a clever framing tactic" was employed by Compassion & Choices to manipulate the presentation of this good showing for political purposes. Maynard's response to this last accusation has already been noted. But again, what she omits in her story is neither a denial of the problems being raised nor an argument against their being solved. She is telling *her* story about the health of *her* lived body, which does not obligate her to offer a more comprehensive assessment of the benefits and burdens of the medical-aid-in-dying movement.

I think it is fair, however, to admit that Compassion & Choices acted strategically in helping to enhance the effectiveness of what Maynard has to say about her situation. For example, in a video recorded on October 13, 2014, Maynard details the development of her brain cancer and her ordeal in having to deal with its consequences. The presentation is delivered in plain-style eloquence. No pictures are shown of her pre-cancer appearance. A perspective by incongruity had already made its mark on what cancer was doing to her lived body. "I am heartbroken that I had to leave behind my home, my community, my friends in California, but I am dying and I refuse to lose my dignity. I refuse to subject myself and my family to purposeless, prolonged pain and suffering at the hands of an incurable disease. . . . And I am preparing to experience the best possible death. Achieving some control over my passing is very important to me. . . . How dare the government make decisions or limit options for terminally ill people like me. The laws in California and 45 other states must change."[45]

The video was first shown to the California Senate Health Committee on March 31, 2015, hours before the committee began debating Senate Bill (SB) 128: "The End of Life Option Act." The bill passed. The five-month delay in showing the video was certainly strategic. I do not believe, however, that the strategy was unethical. Rather, it was a rhetorical maneuver that ensured a face-to-face encounter between the committee and a wounded storyteller whose narrative represented the new face of the movement. The right to design legal strategies that allow your voice to be acknowledged by people in power should not be discouraged by those who oppose what you have to say.

Whether one agrees with them or not, those like Peace and Ellis deserve credit for trying to determine how the rhetorical construction of the new face of the medical-aid-in-dying movement should be received by the public. Their responses to Maynard's story align them with advocates of the right-to-life movement and its goals of blemishing this face of a wounded storyteller. I thus suspect that Peace and Ellis would deny what supporters of Maynard affirm: She was a brave, courageous, and heroic individual.[46] Having a hero become the new face of the medical-aid-in-dying movement adds much to its credibility in making a good showing of a bad situation. A hero embodies the virtues of courage, dignity, and moral integrity. In countering this possibility, advocates of the right-to-life movement advance a notion of heroism that they maintain discredits Maynard's heroic status. The debate over this matter is intense, elevating the role played by the right-to-life movement in its opposition to Maynard's story.

Emmanuel Levinas tells us what a hero is: "Prior to death there is always a last chance; this is what heroes seize, not death. The hero is the one who always glimpses a last chance, the one who obstinately finds chances."[47] This definition accords with Levinas's philosophy of how the other is the basis of ethics and thus how the self has an obligation to respond to the other's presence, especially when the other is in need of help. Recall that Levinas likens the self's obliging relationship with the other to the relationship that forms between God and Adam when God asks, "Where art thou?" and Adam answers, "Here I am!"[48] The hero serves the other. When circumstances threaten that the end is near, the would-be hero searches for a "last chance" to live *for,* and perhaps die *for,* the other.

I think it is fair to say that Maynard acted heroically. She used her last chance at life to live for others. Evidence supporting this claim is found throughout her story. In a video recorded shortly before she died, she makes sure that others know what her purpose is: that of a wounded storyteller. The video was not released until November 19, 2014, as part of a celebration of her thirtieth birthday. I assume that the strategy here was to keep her heroic status alive given the responses from those who would deny her this status.

> I decided to share my story because I felt like this issue of death with dignity is misunderstood by many people in our community and culture and I really wanted people to understand that as I went through the process of being approved for death with dignity that I felt very valued by my physicians here and very protected. There is no way that I could possibly have been coerced into this. It's not a fear based choice, it is a logic based choice. . . . If I can play even the smallest part in helping to reduce fear in our misunderstanding, then it is worth thinking, speaking up for. . . . If there is one message to come away with from everything that I have been through, it is no matter what life kind of presents you with, never be afraid to use your own voice. Even if you are uncertain, even if your voice is shaking, ask the questions you want to ask. Speak up for yourself. Advocate.[49]

Maynard sounds a call of conscience. She wants others to do the same. In the final words she wrote on Facebook right before she died, she had this to say to all those who had acknowledged and assisted in advancing her cause: "Goodbye to all my dear friends and family that I love. Today is the day I have chosen to pass away with dignity in the face of my terminal illness, this terrible brain cancer that has taken so much from me . . . but would have taken so much more. The world is a beautiful place. . . . I even have a ring of support around my bed as I type. . . . Goodbye world. Spread good energy. Pay it forward!"[50]

These final words are significant in evaluating Maynard's heroic status. The fact that the last testament of the new face for medical aid in dying was encountered through social media is significant. Sharing her final message to the world through Facebook makes Maynard a hero for a digital-media generation. Unlike in past high-profile cases, Maynard communicated her last wishes directly to the public. Her last chance to serve others was now complete. But all along she was also serving herself by ending the struggle with the "terrible brain cancer that has taken so much from me" and that "would have taken so much more." I do not fault her for making this decision. The question that now must be asked, however, is this: If a hero is one who seizes a last chance to serve others, can she still be considered a hero if, at the same time, her actions are inextricably tied to a concern for herself?

Critical responses to Maynard from right-to-life advocates focus on her self-interest. By taking her to task for choosing the option of death with dignity, they discredit the basis of her heroic status as a wounded storyteller who has seized her last chance to serve others. So, for example, we have this common response from Truth Teller: "Brittany Maynard was a coward. That isn't an insult. That describes her for what she was. . . . Brittany didn't know the meaning of [dignity]. Dignity means respect. Respect honors achievement. She certainly did not achieve anything except a way out of courage. For she had none of that. She's a rotten example of dignity. . . . We don't have the ability to create a life. We can do the work. But only GOD can create a life. And it is not up to us to end ours. There are very few ways to leave this world with dignity. And that would likely require some real courage to face trials and tribulations to the end. Brittany Maynard faced nothing. She fell backwards."[51]

Two consecutive responses to Truth Teller make clear how contentious and mean-spirited the debate over Maynard's heroic status can be:

> She was an incredibly courageous, brave young woman who made a conscious decision to exercise the ultimate in self-determination—ending her life, when it was no longer worth living (and yes, each and every one of us has the right to make that decision) she had nothing lying ahead of her but debilitation, agony and running her family into bankruptcy. She did the right thing, the cowardly thing is to lay there in pain waiting for "nature to take its course." On one hand I hope you never face a situation like that, and on the other hand—well I'm sorry, but I hope you do.
>
> --
>
> You did not read one word this man wrote . . . because God has blinded you to the truth. . . . If you believe this coward was a hero than you are a very sick man. May God have mercy on you. Your life is always worth living but obviously yours is not. . . . If I or this poster are ever faced with this WE KNOW what we will do and we know what you will do . . . take the evil satanic coward's way out. . . . Satan has many advocates and you are one.

Notice that Truth Teller's response is based on a standard meaning of dignity: respect. (S)he associates this meaning with "achievement," especially as it relates to God. Supporters of the right to life appeal to God when they argue that it takes "real courage to face trials and tribulations to the end." That's achievement. That's respecting God's will. That's demonstrating moral integrity. That's heroic. Another proper meaning of dignity is "self-respect." This meaning is implied in the first response to Truth Teller. Here no reference to God is required. Implied in the second response is the meaning of dignity that Truth Teller emphasizes. A hero demonstrates respect for God. As its Latin root *dignitas* suggests, dignity also means "worthiness," "elevation," "excellence," and "virtue." I suspect that all of these definitions could be used by the respondents to make their points. The meaning of dignity is suitable for both those who support the right to life and those who support the right to die. However, when God is called on to make a decision about the proper meaning and use of the term, advantage goes to the right to life. Indeed, how is one supposed to argue with God? The second response to Truth Teller tells us the fate of those who make an attempt: Satan awaits you. Moses accepted the task and persuaded God not to annihilate the Jewish people when they broke the Law. I think it is fair to say that Moses is not in the company of Satan.

How certain one can be about the correctness of what supporters of the right to life have to say about dignity, God, and heroism is debatable. Indeed, the interruption that we are is ever present with its question: Are you sure? Maynard never mentions God in telling her story, and, as far as I know, the rhetoric of the death-with-dignity movement also has nothing to say about the matter. My references to Maynard's story indicate that her definition of dignity is associated with self-respect and a respect for others—her family and those members of the public that may benefit from her story. As a wounded storyteller, she is living for others until she dies, and afterwards, too. It's a good ending for all concerned, unless you favor the meaning of dignity emphasized by supporters of the right-to-life movement.

Maynard's good ending is what makes her a coward in the eyes of her critics. Her story is first and foremost grounded in self-interest: She does not want to experience the inevitable and unbearable pain and suffering that are bound to happen as her brain cancer takes its full effect on her body and mind. That would not be a good ending to her story, a good showing of a bad situation. Medical aid in dying produces a more favorable outcome. Dying with dignity is a good ending. In voicing their objection to this argument, Maynard's critics promote the counterargument that the new face of the medical-aid-in-dying movement is unworthy of admiration and respect; it lacks moral integrity. Siding with this argument can produce harsh criticism of Maynard's story. The late Kara Tippetts, a hero of the right-to-life movement, believed that such criticism is not the way to go. Tippetts offers a caring and loving response to Maynard—one hero reaching out to another hero. The event became world-wide news with the help of social media. Tippetts's gesture marked a rare moment in the unfolding of

Maynard's story. Her narrative and the public moral argument it informs were now challenged in an unexpected way.

Tippetts had terminal breast cancer. She suffered from the illness for three years. Surgery, chemotherapy, and radiation treatments proved unsuccessful. She passed away on March 22, 2015. She was thirty-eight years old. She left behind a husband and four young children. She approached death with great respect for God. She died with dignity, never giving in to all the pain and suffering caused by her illness. On October 8, 2014, she wrote an "open letter" to Maynard intended to quell the harsh criticism that was and would be clouding a heartfelt understanding of what heroism entails: becoming one with Jesus Christ. The letter was posted on her website and went viral. The website contains a video and photographs that show Tippetts's physical appearance before and after cancer had devastated her body.[52] We see her dying in her bed, withstanding the misery of her condition. The perspective by incongruity employed in the Maynard videos to generate sadness functions in the Tippetts website and video to produce not only that emotion but also joy. Tippetts claims that the agony of dying from cancer can be a beautiful and educational experience for oneself and others when one's dying is aided by an everlasting belief in Christ. Tippetts is a wounded storyteller.

Turning to Christ for assistance in dying is the major theme of her letter. In developing this theme, Tippetts offers the kindest and most compassionate response to Maynard that I found in my research. There is no attempt to denigrate Maynard's character or actions. The word "coward" is never used. Rather, Tippetts emphasizes how her "heart ached" over Maynard's plight. She "prayed [Maynard] would hear [her] words from the most tender and beautifully broken place in [her] Heart." The term "heart" is used eleven times in her letter. To borrow a construct from Kenneth Burke, the "heart" is a "God term" in the rhetoric of the right-to-life movement.[53] Recall that the Bible speaks of conscience in terms of the heart: "I will give them a heart to know me, that I am the Lord" (Jeremiah 24:7). Tippetts's prose not only comes from the heart but is meant to reach the heart. "Knowing what it is to know the horizon of your days that once felt limitless [but that now feel] to be dimming. . . . Brittany, your life matters, your story matters, and your suffering matters. Thank you for stepping out from the privacy of your story and sharing it openly."

Tippetts appreciates the importance of rhetorical eloquence. She employs plain and gracious prose, and everything that she says reflects what she sincerely considers to be the truth that manifests itself in her knowing-with God. This is not to say, however, that Tippetts's loving kindness would have her acknowledge to at least some small degree the heroism of Maynard's actions. "Walk before me and be thou perfect." Tippetts certainly did not see Maynard following this holy command. Which means what exactly? The Bible doesn't say. The command is ambiguous. Tippetts faults Maynard without indicating in no uncertain terms that she knows for sure what the definition of perfection truly is. Still, Tippetts sounds a call of conscience intended to direct Maynard toward a more perfect way of being. Tippetts has a problem that she refuses to acknowledge.

But Tippetts is persistent. The key is getting Maynard to appreciate the value of suffering, which the rhetoric of the medical-aid-in-dying movement refuses to recognize. Tippetts tells Maynard that "there are countless lovers of your heart that are praying that you would change your mind [about the matter]. Suffering is not the absence of goodness, it is not the absence of beauty." Tippetts's words reflect her understanding of and commitment to the teachings of her Savior. These teachings stress the importance of instructions associated with this Savior's religious heritage: "Where art thou? Here I am!"; "Choose life," not death (Deuteronomy 30:19). We owe God acknowledgment. Suffering should not be a reason for Maynard to commit what the rhetoric of the right to life labels "the sin" of suicide. Tippetts never uses the word sin in her letter. That is too harsh of a term for Tippetts's purposes, although she does use the word "suicide" in the title of her letter. As noted earlier, Maynard stresses that the term has no application to her story; suggesting that it does is offensive.

Tippet never again mentions the term. Rather, she finds a more eloquent way of referring to the act in question and its consequences: "In choosing your own death, you are robbing those that love you with such tenderness the opportunity of meeting you in your last moments and extending your love in your last breaths. . . . That last kiss, that last warm touch, that last breath, matters—but it was never intended for us to decide when that last breath is breathed." No, the time of death is up to God. Tippetts refers to her upcoming death from cancer to emphasize the beauty of it all:

> Knowing Jesus, knowing that He understands my hard goodbye, He walks with me in my dying. My heart longs for you to know Him in your dying. Because in his dying, he protected my living. . . . Brittany, when we trust Jesus to be the carrier, protector, redeemer of our hearts, death is no longer dying. . . . You have been told a lie. A horrible lie, that your dying will not be beautiful. That suffering will be too great. . . . But in my whisper, pleading, loving voice dear heart—will you hear my heart ask you, beg you, plead with you—not to take that pill. Yes, your dying will be hard, but it will not be without beauty. . . . I pray that my words reach you. I pray they reach the multitudes that are looking at your story and believing the lie that suffering is a mistake, that dying isn't to be braved, that choosing our death is the courageous story.

Tippetts longs for Maynard to be heroic. Christ is here to ensure that the challenge will be worth the struggle, pain, and suffering. There is beauty to behold in meeting this challenge. The beauty shows itself as Tippetts serves others by allowing them to witness her dying moments, acknowledge how much she means to them, and thereby demonstrate the same virtue that Tippetts displays in her suffering presence: the ethical duty of living *for* others. For those who believe in all that she has to say in her letter to Maynard, Tippetts is a hero for would-be heroes. She did everything required to be acknowledged as such. She seized the opportunity of a last chance to live for others, right up to the very end. Her dignity is undeniable, as is her moral integrity. She practiced what she preached. And what she preached in her letter to Maynard showed compassion and what it means to have a heart for those who oppose your beliefs regarding matters of life and death. Tippetts set a standard of civility for critics of Maynard's story. That is what makes her letter so special. Although I am not a follower of the religious orientation that informs Tippetts's plea, I respect her effort in reaching out to another wounded storyteller. But I also am troubled by her use of a term contained in the last quotation cited earlier.

Tippetts tells Maynard three times that she has been told a "lie" about the worthlessness of suffering. Given that Maynard is promoting that supposed lie with her story, Maynard qualifies as also being a liar. I know of no Scripture that commands someone to tell a person who is near death and suffering from the physical and psychological consequences of her illness that she should be called a liar. Where's the compassion? Have a "heart"! The same could be said for the right-to-life movement as a whole, claiming a moral high ground while calling a dying woman a liar who misunderstands the worth of her own life and suffering.

Whether she realizes it or not, Tippetts is being harsh with her kindness, and this is especially so if, to alleviate her own suffering, she is taking medication for her pain, which is never revealed nor denied. Her belief in the sanctity of life and the normative positions surrounding stewardship and the transcendent meaning of suffering are no longer lessons to impart but rather an exercise in proselytizing. Given the unquestioned ideology that she is abiding by, how does Tippetts know for sure that she herself is not a liar? EddieInCA, a commenter on an article about Tippetts's criticism of Maynard, puts it this way: "If I were in the position of Brittany Maynard, and made the decision after careful consult with my wife, doctors, parents, and anyone else I cared about, and then received this sort of proselytizing, I'd be offended. Heck, I'm not Brittany Maynard and I'm offended. How effin' dare Kara Tippets [*sic*] think that her way is 'better' than that of Brittany Maynard? Why? Because she's religious?"[54]

Maynard's convictions were too strong to be influenced by Tippetts's letter. It is important to realize, however, that Maynard's definition of dignity and the good death it allows does not prohibit Tippetts from dying the good death that she values and thus being the hero that her supporters claim that she is.

Tippetts's definition of dignity, however, does prohibit Maynard from dying the good death that she values and having the heroic status that her supporters praise. This lack of reciprocity seems a bit unfair. Reciprocity, however, can be achieved while still allowing Tippetts to die her good death. Maynard would have had to persuade Tippetts and her supporters to allow for some flexibility in their interpretation of God's good will. If she had any chance of being successful, Maynard would have been wise to include a positive reference to God in her endeavor. For example: Tippetts tells us that, owing to God's assistance, a person with terminal cancer can experience beauty in the unbearable pain and suffering caused by the illness. For advocates of the death-with-dignity movement, unbearable suffering qualifies as a "living death." Do you think God is gracious enough to see a limit to unbearable suffering and thereby admit that the command "Choose life, not death" disqualifies a living death as being life? If so, then avoiding a living death should qualify as seizing a last chance to act in a virtuous manner. Perhaps this way of thinking about the matter at hand is what is needed to abide by the command "Walk before me and be thou perfect." A good death adds a last bit of goodness to the good life.

I believe that this attempt to reason with Tippetts and her supporters is worth considering, if only to determine how much credit they grant God for being what they claim God is: Gracious! I also believe that Maynard would not have been interested in conducting the inquiry. She didn't need the support of her critics to die with dignity. She refused to accept that she was victimized by some horrible lie about the value of suffering. She was not afraid of dying. She did not believe that self-interest disqualified the authenticity of how she used the death sentence of her illness to live for others. Critics of Tippetts could say there was also self-interest in her case. All that she said and did served her desire to be acknowledged as a devout Christian. Tippetts and her supporters would undoubtedly take great exception to this charge. Maynard and her supporters would likely respond in kind. How she put a last chance to use was brave, courageous, and heroic. Maynard, too, is a hero for would-be heroes. Tippetts and her supporters would have an obvious response: You have an ungodly understanding of what qualifies as a last chance and a good death. Tippetts probably would have toned down the harshness of the accusation. Maynard, too. Nothing she has to say in telling her story is voiced in a harsh way. She never demeans her critics. Even when she takes exception to the accusation that she is planning to commit the heinous act of suicide, Maynard goes only as far as to make a claim that I quoted earlier: "I am not suicidal. If I were, I would have consumed that medication long ago. I do not want to die. But I am dying." Maynard's critics remain oblivious to this obvious point; hence the claim by the psychologist Steven Ertelt that Maynard's death was "the most public suicide of modern history."[55]

Like Tippetts, Maynard sets a standard of civility for those whose reactions to her story are far too unfitting in tone. Civility, unfortunately, will not be enough to remedy the differences that separate those who favor the medical-aid-in-dying movement and those who do not. What stands in the way is a reified understanding of God's will, held by true believers on one side of the debate and the strongly held conviction by their opposition that God's will (whatever that is, if anything at all) has nothing to do with the matter at hand. And, so, public moral argument goes on about what counts as a dignified way to die a good death.

Conclusion

We must remember that opposing sides on the subject of death have no experience of what it means to be a hero-in-death; otherwise they would be too dead to share their story. For Maynard, Tippetts, and everyone in between, the only common experiences are with living with suffering but never about one's actual death. There is no finalized truth on what it means to be a hero-in-death. Hardcore, unbending belief in religious doctrine stands in the way of reconciliation, refusing the possibility that God is more benevolent and gracious than such belief insists is the case. There are, however, exceptions to the rule.

One day after Tippetts posted her letter to Maynard, Jessica Kelly, a self-described "Christ follower," offered an extensive, well-written, heartfelt, and respectful response to Tippetts.[56] Kelly tells the story of her four-year old son, who died from brain cancer. She details the agony she and her husband went through as they cared for their suffering child. The situation was brutal. Kelly then explains, contra Tippetts, why death is not beautiful, dying is not devoid of courage, and God does not control death. In ending her response, Kelly addresses Maynard: "Brittany—if you read this, please know that as a Christ-follower, I honor your choice. If I were in your shoes, it would be my choice as well. It would grant me incredible emotional freedom to enjoy the days I face, and to make the most of them. I believe God is by your side. I see tremendous love, courage, and beauty in your eyes. Thank you for sharing your story."

Maynard's story functions rhetorically and virtuously with its commitment to the authenticity of self-determination, living for others, dignity, moral integrity, eloquence, sincerity, and offering a narrative that helps to legitimate the heroic character of a wounded storyteller, despite this teller's self-interest in wanting to die with dignity. Kelly was moved by Maynard's story in its early development. That's something that rhetoric is supposed to do. Admitting that both Tippetts and Maynard possess moral integrity, Kelly ends her response to these wounded storytellers with a wish: "As we discuss these issues together, my greatest prayer is for gentle tones and ready ears."

Kelly's wish lends support to my earlier stated belief that an open-minded conversation between supporters of the right to die and advocates of the right to life about the extent of God's graciousness would be worthwhile. The interruption that we are calls for such conversation and the arguments that go with it. And let us not forget the virtues that mark this communicative and rhetorical activity and that contribute to the good health of the lived body: self-determination, wholeheartedness, conscience, eloquence, listening, respect, dignity, moral integrity, considerateness, forbearance, tolerance, and intellectual generosity. There is a lot to lose when we become forgetful of what is called for by the interruption that we are. Of course, sooner or later there comes a time when being resolute and taking a stand on some contested issue makes good sense. The perfective impulse of the interruption that we are will nevertheless remain active, always challenging us with a question: Are you sure? An essential feature of existence keeps us honest—another virtue to add to the list.

Owing to the unlikelihood that supporters and critics of Maynard and Tippetts will agree to have the open-minded conversation called for by the interruption that we are, I suspect that right-to-die advocates will continue denying the need to seek God's advice on the proper way to die. Offended by this dismissal of their guiding light, right-to-life supporters will continue to disparage their opposition, making it harder for those like Maynard to get all fifty states to legalize aid in dying.[57] More wounded storytellers supporting the right to die are bound to appear on the national scene. Right-to-life supporters will continue to use harsh and tempered rhetoric to voice their disapproval. And all of this being the case, I have come to the following conclusion: The rhetorical construction of the new face of the medical-aid-in-dying movement will never be without those who are dedicated to calling into question, if not denigrating, the story of Brittany Maynard, which forms the presence of this face. These actions are meant to ensure that the face is flawed, far from perfect. Maynard's story leads me to believe that these actions have achieved slim success. I think it is fair to say that as it currently exists, the story and its face will continue to make a good showing of a bad situation. Are you sure?

I am sure that Maynard would agree with my conclusion. I am also sure that Tippetts would not. Maynard's decision is based totally on personal and legal rights. Tippetts's decision is based totally on what she understands to be God's authority. "Walk before me and be thou perfect." Without knowing what perfection means, how does Tippetts know that Maynard's way of walking is not applauded by God? Perfection is as elusive as it is worth pursuing. The perfective impulse of the interruption that we are speaks to us of the importance of the endeavor. More than the case studies examined so far, the next one has much to tell us about the benefits and burdens associated with the task at hand. The health and good life of our lived bodies are on the line.

CHAPTER 7

Our Posthuman Future

> "The best possible time to contest for what the posthuman means is now, before the trains of thought it embodies have been laid down so firmly that it would take dynamite to change them."
>
> N. Katherine Hayles, *How We Became Posthuman*

Imagine you are Charles Siebert, who has inherited his father's heart disease, or William Schroeder, connected to his Jarvik-7, or Harriet McBryde Johnson, whose degenerative neuromuscular disease requires that she be lifted from her bed every day and put in a wheelchair, or the parent of an infant who is severely disabled with no chance of qualifying as a person, or Brittany Maynard or Kara Tippetts, both dying from terminal cancer. How would you respond to the following inquiry issued by the President's Council on Bioethics (PCB) during its deliberations on the topic "Biotechnology and the Pursuit of Happiness"? Keep in mind that a mandate of the PCB is to generate deliberation and public moral argument about contested issues in bioethics and to use "fair and accurate terminology" in defining these issues:

> Seemingly from the beginning, human beings have been alive to the many ways in which what we have been given falls short of what we can envision and what we desire. We are human, but can imagine gods. We die, but can imagine immortality. . . . Although [human beings] are far from omnipotent, we have extraordinary powers, unique among the earth's creatures, to shape our environments and even ourselves according to our wills. It is perhaps not surprising, therefore that also from the beginning human beings have struggled with two opposing responses to our lot. Should we try to mold the imperfection we have been given into something closer to our ideal? Or should we content ourselves with beholding and enjoying it as it is? And what about our own natures? Does our ability to flourish as human beings depend on our ability to improve upon the human form or

function? Or might the contrary be true: does our flourishing depend on accepting—or even celebrating—our natural limitations?[1]

If you favor the first option in each of the two pairs of questions, you are siding with the perspective of posthumanity, also referred to as transhumanism. If you favor the second option in each of the two pairs of questions, you are siding with the perspective of bioconservatism. Before you make an informed decision, another question must be addressed: What do bioconservatives mean by "natural limitations"?

A basic answer to the question is this: those physical and mental attributes that people are gifted with by nature. The quality of this gift can be alarming. As Leon Kass, a leading bioconservative and one-time chairperson of the PCB, points out, "When Nature deals her cards, some receive only from the bottom of the deck."[2] So, for example, natural limitations are on display in the genetically influenced lived bodies of Siebert, his father, Schroeder, Johnson, severely disabled infants, Maynard, and Tippetts. However, before the lived body receives its gift from nature, another gift, another natural limitation, has already been given: the interruption that we are. From an existential point of view, this gift is the most fundamental one that there is. Indeed, it was present before anybody emerged from his or her mother's womb. What makes this gift so special is its perfective impulse, which calls for concerned thought and action, self-determination, moral responsibility, the fortitude that is needed to improve one's situation in life and to feel more complete as a person, and the rhetorical competence to spread the word as a way of helping others in need. In short, the perfective impulse of the interruption that we are calls people to be as perfect as they can be no matter how close to the bottom of the deck they are. The alternative is falling victim to the interruption's defeatist impulse

Bioconservatives are supportive of the endeavor to improve the health of the lived body, up to a point. They expect medicine to employ its biotechnologies to cure illness whenever possible and to provide therapeutic assistance when caring for those whose illnesses cannot be cured, but these practices must not go beyond "our natural limitations." Whose natural limitations? The person who is ill? Why not the natural limitations of a world-class athlete? In order for the ill person, once cured, to achieve that level of excellence, the person might decide to use steroids and other drugs to enhance his or her physical and mental stamina. Bioconservatives see such enhancement as disrespecting the normative standard of our natural limitations, which should direct the curative and therapeutic goals of medicine.[3] Enhancement, they say, places us on a slippery slope leading to an unbridled use of biotechnology to recreate and improperly "master" the nature of human being.[4] Such is the way of posthumanity, argue bioconservatives, and the consequences are likely to be troubling. Kass offers this description of the situation: "Human nature itself lies on the operating table, ready for alteration, for eugenic and psychic 'enhancement,' for wholesale redesign. In leading laboratories new creators are confidently amassing their powers and quietly honing their skills, while on the street their evangelists are zealously prophesying a post-human future. For anyone who cares about preserving our humanity, the time has come to pay attention."[5]

The fear appeal is obvious, although it pales in comparison when the philosopher and bioethicist George Annas and his coauthors Lori Andrews and Rosario Isasi have their say: "The new species, or 'posthuman,' will likely view the old 'normal' humans as inferior, even savages, and fit for slavery or slaughter. The normal, on the other hand, may see the posthumans as a threat and if they can, may engage in a preemptive strike by killing the posthumans before they themselves are killed or enslaved by them." According to Annas and his coauthors, such a result constitutes a "crime against humanity." They therefore contend that "it is ultimately this predictable potential for genocide that makes species-altering experiments potential weapons of mass destruction, and makes the unaccountable genetic engineer a potential bioterrorist."[6]

Bioconservatives give enhancement a bad name. In so doing, they are open to the charge that they lack a fair and accurate understanding of the phenomenon. The philosopher Allen Buchanan refers to the life of the scientist to correct this problem: "Each individual scientist is cognitively enhanced through a long and demanding period of education and training. . . . The expertise of individual scientists is employed in a set of practices that define the community of scientists. This community is not only international; it's also intergenerational. Taken together, the scientific community's practices for knowledge-seeking constitute a brilliant collective of cognitive enhancement."[7]

The bioethicist Arthur Caplan offers a more expansive response to the problem: "[Bioconservatives] suggest that if we start to muck around at improving and enhancing ourselves, we're going to become 'posthuman.' This argument about what we can or cannot do to design ourselves is made by people who wear eyeglasses, use insulin, have artificial hips or heart values, profit from tissue or organ transplants, ride on airplanes, talk on phones, and sit under electric lights. What are they talking about? Are we posthuman if we ride but don't walk? We might be less healthy but posthuman? I don't see an argument here that says there's a natural boundary or limit that tells us that our nature is defiled by technology."[8]

The award-winning science journalist writer Ronald Bailey has this to say about the matter when discussing what he terms "liberation biology." Such liberation, writes Bailey, "began when the first human sharpened a stick and used it to kill an animal for food. Further liberation from biological constraints followed with fire, the wheel, domesticating animals, agriculture, metallurgy, city building, textiles, information storage by means of writing, the internal combustion engine, electric power generation, antibiotics, vaccines, transplants, and contraception. In a sense, *the* goal toward which humanity has been striving for millennia has been to liberate ourselves, by extending our capacities, from more and more of our ancestors' biological constraints."

Indeed, quips Bailey, "It's not as though most of us still live in our species' 'natural state' as Pleistocene hunter-gathers."[9] The microbiologist Lee Silver also has a wonderful way of addressing the issue: "Air conditioners, airplanes, antibiotics, automobiles, cameras, computers, cyberspace, firework displays, food preservatives, genetic engineering, the Global Positioning System for Navigation, iPods, in vitro fertilization, microscopes, MRI scans, radios, refrigerators, rockets, remote-control rovers on Mars, space probes build by humans leaving the solar system, glass-and-steel skyscrapers, telephones, telescopes, television, vaccines, and a multitude of other Promethean biological, chemical, and physical technologies would all have seemed like magic if they had been described to the most educated people of generations past. In the future as well, no doubt, magic will happen and humankind will self-evolve."[10]

Buchanan, Caplan, Bailey, and Silver return us to the issue of our natural limitations. How is one to know for sure that this gift should dictate the boundaries for the proper use of biotechnology? Kass turns to the Bible to answer the question, for here we learn, as Kass puts it, that "God is concerned with the goodness or perfection of things."[11] Indeed, "Walk before me and be thou perfect." Presumably, Kass, like Tippetts, knows what God means by "perfection," although Kass, unlike Tippetts, does not leave us guessing. Perfection is defined by humankind's natural limitations! But God never says that. The meaning of perfection remains ambiguous. It's a rhetorical maneuver that interrupts the certainty of our common sense and encourages public moral argument. God is the master rhetorician. Goodness is perfection in the making. Given Kass's religious based claim about our natural limitations, the journey is over. Humankind is now as perfect as it should be.[12] Another gift, that might be related to God—the interruption that we are, with its perfective impulse—is always here to call into question Kass's bold claim: Are you sure? Are you sure? Are you sure? "Walk before me and be thou perfect" might be a command instructing humankind to improve upon the human form or function as it was long ago and still is.

I can't imagine people like Siebert, his father, Schroeder, Johnson, parents of severely disabled infants, Maynard, and even Tippetts would not hope for the best. Posthumanists share this hope. Bailey notes: "Nobody said the future would be risk free and the moral choices easy, but the future also brings wondrous new opportunities to cure disease, alleviate suffering, end hunger and lengthen healthy lives. We would be less than human not to seize those opportunities."[13] Elsewhere Bailey writes: "People who take advantage of the fruits of biotechnological progress in the future will be neither Frankenstein monsters nor genetic robots. Rather, they will be our grateful descendants for whom we have eased the burden of disease, disability, and early death, if only we choose not to slow or kill the development of this new technology. They will look back in wonder, and perhaps in horror, at those who would have denied them the blessings of biomedical progress.[14] The award-winning author and bioethicist Gregory Stock adds to this hopeful look of posthumanity: "We know that *Homo sapiens* is not the final word in primate evolution, but few have yet grasped that we are on the cusp of profound biological change, poised to transcend our current form and character on a journey to destinations of new imagination. . . . Some imagine we will see the perils, come to our senses, and turn away from such possibilities. But when we imagine Prometheus stealing fire from the gods, we are not incredulous or shocked by his act. It is too characteristically human. To forgo the powerful technologies that genomics and molecular biology are bringing would be as out of character for humanity as it would be to use them without concern for the dangers they pose. We will do neither."[15]

One reason that this balanced approach will be maintained is that scientists will remain true to the call of the interruption that we are, make good use of its perfective impulse, acknowledge the legitimacy of its question "Are you sure?," and engage in the rhetorical activity of public moral argument so to defend and, whenever necessary, amend the declared truthfulness of their claims regarding our postmodern future. Dr. Francis Collins, who led the team that discovered the language of the human genome, favors the practice of this process. His discovery serves as a major catalyst in fostering public moral argument about the benefits and burdens of posthumanity. With this discovery, Collins came to the conclusion that responding to the call of the interruption that we are requires that one additional factor be accepted in order to account for the ability of scientists to offer a wholehearted response. Evidence of this factor is present in the language of the human genome. For this language, according to Collins, is, in fact, the "language of God," the One who gifted us with the Moral Law that we embody and that enables us to determine right from wrong. (Speak about making perfect use of the perfectionist impulse of language.) In a lecture presented at the University of California, Berkeley, in 2008, Collins offered a series of slides that summarized his thinking on the creation of the Moral Law: Slide 1: "Almighty God, who is not limited in space or time, created a universe 13.7 billion years ago with its parameters precisely tuned to allow the development of complexity over long periods of time." Slide 2: "God's plan included the mechanism of evolution to create the marvelous diversity of living things on our planet. Most especially, that creative plan included human beings." Slide 3: "After evolution had prepared a sufficiently advanced 'house' (the human brain), God gifted humanity with the knowledge of good and evil (the Moral Law), with free will, and with an immortal soul. Slide 4: "We humans use our free will to break the Moral Law, leading to our estrangement from God. For Christians, Jesus is the solution to that estrangement." Slide 5: "If the Moral Law is just a side effect of evolution, then there is no such thing as good or evil. It's all an illusion. We've been hoodwinked. Are any of us, especially the strong atheists, really prepared to live our lives within this worldview?"[16]

Collins tells the story of how he came to know and celebrate the Moral Law in his book *The Language of God*. The story is also shared and developed in a host of public presentations and interviews. The story is rightly seen as an instance of public moral argument emphasizing the way science and religion, in his opinion, are necessarily related. My discussion of this story is in line with the way I read and commented on the previous three stories. I use Collins's story as a bridge to various other instances of public moral argument involved in the debate over our posthuman future. What I have to say about this debate is not intended to be comprehensive. The points I emphasize primarily serve the purpose of keeping my story going about the interruption that we are and its relationship to the health of the lived body and the rhetorical construction of narratives in public moral argument.

Francis Collins and Others

Collins was once an atheist. He was twenty-two. His training in and devotion to science situated him comfortably in this profession's world of know-how, with its disciplined understanding of the logical workings of reason and empiricism. In this world, there is no doubt that God is a myth. As time went on and extended conversations with associates about "belief" took place, Collins found himself "with a combination of willful blindness and something that could only be properly described as arrogance, having avoided any serious consideration that God might be a real possibility. Suddenly all my arguments [for dismissing God] seemed very thin. And I had the sensation that the ice under my feet was cracking. This realization was a thoroughly terrifying experience."[17] Stated another way, Collins's secure world of know-how had been interrupted and dismantled enough that he became exposed to the interruption that we are. The anxiety produced by this exposure can, indeed, be a terrifying experience. Collins found himself caught up in the tension between the interruption's defeatist impulse and its perfective impulse. The rhetorical construction of a narrative that could relieve the tension was desperately needed. The health of Collins's lived body depended on it. The perfective impulse was put into play. The narrative was already partially at hand. Collins accepted Jesus Christ as his personal savior, while still holding on to the wonders of science. And so he tells us:

"Science's domain is to explore nature. God's domain is in the spiritual world, a realm not possible to explore with the tools and language of science. It must be examined with the heart, the mind, and the soul—and the mind must find a way to embrace both realms" (6). Collins now inhabited a new and exceedingly virtuous world of know-how. Here one can learn much about the importance of being compassionate, respectful, a person of dignity and moral integrity, and a person who is courageous enough to engage in the heroic struggle of fighting for the good of humanity. Collins has nothing to say about the matter.

In June 2000, it was announced that a rough draft of the language of the human genome was complete. The human genome—the complete set of human genes—consists of all the DNA of our species, the hereditary code of life. Its language forms a text that is three billion letters long. Collins tells us that during a White House East Room gathering celebrating the momentous scientific achievement, President Clinton compared the map of the human genome to the map of our country that the "frontier" explorer Meriwether Lewis unfolded before President Thomas Jefferson two hundred years earlier in the same room of state. "Without a doubt," claimed Clinton, "this is the most important, must wondrous map ever produced by humankind. . . . Today . . . we are learning the language in which God created life. We are gaining ever more awe for the complexity, the beauty, and the wonder of God's most divine and sacred gift" (2). Collins admits that he helped craft the speech. When it was time for Collins to speak, he made the moment a bit more personal: "It's a happy day for the world. It is humbling for me, and awe-inspiring to realize that we have caught the first glimpse of our own instruction book, previously known only to God" (3). Presumably, this book, given its author, contained all that was needed to ensure, among other things, that human beings had the genetic basis for developing all the virtues that are needed for human beings to flourish as a species.

Collins never deals directly with this issue of virtues. He never tires, however, of repeating how he was awestruck by discovering the language of God. For example: "Evolution, as a mechanism, can be and must be true. But that says nothing about the nature of its author. For those who believe in God, there are reasons now to be more in awe, not less" (107); "This book was written in the DNA language by which God spoke life into being. I felt an overwhelming sense of awe in surveying this most significant of all biological texts" (123–24). "Awe" is a major term in Collins's narrative, which makes sense since the term lies at the heart of the Judeo-Christian narrative. Awe is *the* state of mind that enables a person to acquire some sense that there is such a thing as God. Awe opens a person to the call "Where art thou?" and grants the person an opportunity to say "Here I am!" with all her heart. Without awe, God never comes to mind in all of God's glory. In an age when the term "awesome" is tossed around like a worn-out coin—"Hey, this bowl of Captain Crunch is awesome"—it is all too easy to forget or care less about what the true meaning of awe entails. Have you ever experienced awe? How did you feel? What did you think? What did you say? Did you have the words to capture and disclose all that happened to you? Perhaps you were at a loss for words. Why? Collins never addresses these questions. He never clarifies what awe means and how it works. Given the religious narrative that informs his thinking, he certainly had the directives to do so. For example, he could have noted, as does Rabbi Abraham Heschel, that "*The beginning of awe is wonder, and the beginning of wisdom is awe.*"[18] And he could have added: "Awe . . . is more than a feeling. It is an answer of the heart and mind to the presence of mystery in all things, *an intuition for a meaning that is beyond the mystery, an awareness of the transcendent worth of the universe*" (106). And then he could have added this: "The more eager we are to express [awe], the less remains of it" (75).

Perhaps Collins had this last point in mind when he decided not to expand on his use of the term. And given that he is telling a story intended to encourage public moral argument about his topic but also rhetorically designed for untrained thinkers, he thought that a more elaborate discussion of awe would be too intellectual for his audience. Or perhaps he chose not to do any more than mention the term as a way of limiting attacks from nonbelievers who already had had too much of his "religious nonsense." The attacks, nevertheless, were forthcoming, and they were often harsh. The more brutal came from the neuroscientist, philosopher, and atheist Sam Harris: "*The Language of God* is a genuinely astonishing book. To read it is to witness nothing less than an intellectual suicide. It is, however, a suicide that has gone almost entirely unacknowledged: The body yielded to the rope; the neck snapped; the breath subsided; and the corpse dangles in ghastly discomposure even now—and yet polite people everywhere continue to celebrate the great man's health."[19] Harris's zealous critique of Collins operates at times as if it were composed by a deconstructionist on steroids. For Harris, God is nothing but a fantasy for the weak of mind and heart.

Harris knows that his claims will be shocking to true believers throughout the world. As he sees it, however, the negative reaction to his godless views helps to make clear just how confused his critics are: "Christians generally imagine that no faith imparts the virtues of love and forgiveness more effectively than their own. The truth is that many who claim to be transformed by Christ's love are deeply, even murderously, intolerant of criticism. While we may want to ascribe this to human nature, it is clear that such hatred draws considerable support from the Bible. How do I know this? The most disturbed of my correspondents always cite chapter and verse."[20]

Harris admits that Collins's map warrants high praise for its scientific understanding of life. That the territory supposedly speaks of God's frontier is, however, a mark of ignorance. Hence, as stated in his *Letter to a Christian Nation*,

Harris's goal is "to demolish the intellectual and moral pretensions of Christianity in its most committed forms"—forms that make America appear "like a lumbering, bellicose, dim-witted giant," a country where more than half of its citizens "believe that the entire cosmos was created six thousand years ago." Harris points out that the absurdity of this belief is seen in its conclusion: The Creation occurred "about a thousand years after Sumerians invented glue."[21]

Similar criticism was offered by the evolutionary biologist Richard Dawkins during a debate with Collins, who was explaining how evolution was planned by God and how this plan included the development of human beings endowed with the gift of Moral Law. Dawkins replied: "I think that's a tremendous cop-out. If God wanted to create life and create humans, it would be slightly odd that he should choose the extraordinarily roundabout way of waiting for 10 billion years before life got started and then waiting for another 4 billion years until you got human beings capable of worshipping and sinning and all the other things religious people are interested in." Collins responded: "Who are we to say that that was an odd way to do it? I don't think that it is God's purpose to make his intention absolutely obvious to us. If it suits him to be a deity that we must seek without being forced to, would it not have been sensible for him to use the mechanism of evolution without posting obvious road signs to reveal his role in creation?"[22]

One doesn't have to be religious to experience awe and what it can lead to. Collins never puts any restrictions on the experience. Posthumanists were awed by Collins's discovery and its potential for scientific advances in DNA diagnostic tools, gene-discovery software applications, embryonic cloning procedures, stem cell research, regenerative medicine, organ harvesting and transplantation, genetic engineering, genetic editing—all of which could benefit the goals of human enhancement. Collins offers reassurance to these advances, even if they are not the result of religious belief: "Science is not threatened by God; it is *enhanced*. God is most certainly not threatened by science; He made it all possible" (233, my emphasis). An example of what posthumanists were led to fantasize about with the human genome project in mind is provided by the philosopher and bioethicist Nick Bostrum, director of the Future of Humanity Institute and Oxford University's Program on the Impacts of Future Technology.

> Let us suppose that you were to develop into a being that has posthuman healthspan and posthuman cognitive and emotional capacities. At the early steps of this process [of posthumanity], you enjoy your enhanced capacities. You cherish your improved health; you feel stronger, more energetic, and more balanced. Your skin looks younger and is more elastic. A minor ailment in your knee is cured. You also discover a greater clarity of mind. You can concentrate on difficult material more easily and it begins making

> sense to you. . . . You can follow lines of thinking and intricate argumentation farther without losing your foothold. Your mind is able to recall facts, names, and concepts just when you need them. You are able to sprinkle your conversation with witty remarks and poignant anecdotes. . . . You begin to treasure almost every moment of life; you go about your business with zest; and you feel a deeper warmth and affection for those you love, but you can still be upset and even angry on occasions where upset or anger is truly justified and constructive. . . . You have invented entirely new art forms, which exploit the new kinds of cognitive capacities and sensibilities you have developed. . . . You are communicating with your contemporaries using a language that has grown out of English over the past century and that has a vocabulary and expressive power that enable you to share and discuss thoughts and feelings that unaugmented humans could not even think or experience. . . . You are always ready to feel with those who suffer misfortunes, and to work hard to help them get back on their feet. . . . Things are getting better, but already each day is fantastic.[23]

Bostrum's posthuman dream is meant to be awesome. Some respondents, like the philosopher and bioethics scholar Nicholas Agar, were not impressed. Agar sees this dimension of the narrative as being guilty of "focalism" (that is, people thinking about some intended event in a vacuum, failing to remember that their lived bodies will be affected by many other events that may not have such glorious consequences). According to Agar, "The emotional coloration in [Bostrom's] sales pitch for radical enhancement seems like that for a time share apartment in a tropical spot."[24] Agar takes issue with such hyperbolic rhetoric, for its glorified imaginary outlook makes us forgetful of the "precautionary approach" that should be applied to the use of any medical and biotechnological enhancement. When it comes to this matter and the progress it favors, one should err on the side of caution. Human beings are incapable of knowing all of the variables that have to do with the enactment and consequences of enhancement.[25] And there is a related problem, as well.

Bostrum's vision does not fully account for the dynamics of the interruption that we are. There is no call that would have the self demonstrate the ethical and moral acts of questioning his behavior out of respect for others. Bostrom does note that the self and others could share and discuss thoughts and feelings and that the self would serve others in times of need. But there is no explicit acknowledgment and detailed discussion of how the self would deal with the interruption of others taking exception to the self's purported truth claims. The need for rhetorical competence is basically gone, as are questions of right and wrong.[26] So much for the Moral Law. Indeed, without the interruption that we are, there is no Moral Law to speak of.

Attending to the problems posed by Bostrum's vision, especially as they concern the status of the Moral Law, I suspect Collins might suggest that Bostrum's understanding of awe does not go high enough. I also suspect that, given my last statement about the matter, he would say the same thing to me, and a bit more: Without the One who created the Moral Law, there would be no interruption that we are. Given what I have said about this interruption, there would be a need for further discussion and clarification. The interruption that we are testifies to the importance of transcendence. Still, Collins might find it necessary to turn to the narrative of his religious tradition and state explicitly: "Awe is an intuition for the creaturely dignity of all things and their preciousness to God; a realization that things not only are what they are but also stand, however remotely, for something absolute. Awe is a sense for the transcendence, for the reference everywhere to Him who is beyond all things."[27] But, again, Collins avoids discussing the religious dimensions and workings of awe. His discussion of the phenomenon is antiseptic. He offers but a skeletal version of Christianity. His training as a physician is obvious when he attends to the rhetorical treatment of these topics. Given that religion plays an insignificant role in the narrative of posthumanity, perhaps he is doing posthumanists a favor.

Indeed, Collins is not out to bash these folk as he tells his story about the language of God. Rather, he expresses cautious support for their hope of progress. For example, he notes that "Genetic discoveries and genetic testing will not be dangerous additions to medicine. They will be very valuable once we understand enough about them. But one fear is that we will commit enough egregious errors . . . that the American public will be totally turned off and will decide . . . they don't want anything to do with genetic technology. . . . We don't need a genetic thalidomide."[28] We hear more caution when he discusses the topic of enhancement and asks the question "Who decides what is an 'improvement'?" He continues: "How disastrous might it be to reengineer our species, only to discover we had lost something critical (like resistance to an emerging disease) along the way? And how would such wholesale redesign affect our relationship with our Creator?" (264).

With what has so far been said about the topic of posthumanity, I trust it is clear that these questions are commonplace in evaluating the promises and perils of our posthuman future. The research program of Dr. Anthony Atala (physician, surgeon, and director of Wake Forest Baptist Medical Center's Institute for Regenerative Medicine) is instructive when attempting to answer these questions.[29]

Atala is a leader in the science of tissue engineering, which involves growing organs and tissue in the lab to replace patients' damaged or diseased organs and tissue. The process usually starts with a three-dimensional structure called a scaffold that is used to support cells as they grow and develop. Skin, blood vessels, bladders, trachea, urethras, esophagus, muscle, and other types of tissue have been successfully engineered, and some of these tissues have already been used in treating human disease. Atala was the first scientist to create a laboratory-grown bladder and implant it in a patient. He also led a team of researchers who, between 2005 and 2008, were the first to create laboratory-grown vaginal organs and implant them in four teenage girls who were born with Mayer-Rokitansky-Kuster-Hauser (MRKH) syndrome, a rare genetic condition in which the vagina and uterus are underdeveloped or absent. The organs were engineered with the girls' own cells. Data from annual follow-up examinations showed that even up to eight years after the surgeries, the organs had normal function. In addition, the patients' responses to a Female Sexual Function Index questionnaire showed they also had normal sexual function after the treatment, including desire and painfree intercourse.[30]

This research accomplishment certainly qualifies as an example of science making good use of the perfective impulse of the interruption that we are to improve the health of the lived body. My students, especially the females, describe the accomplishment as "unbelievable" and "awesome." I think these are fair and accurate descriptions of the improvement. To improve something is to enhance its current state of being to a better state of being. In the case of the four teenage girls, the enhancement stayed within the boundaries of a female's natural limitations. Kass should be happy, as should Collins. The "relationship with our Creator" has not been degraded. On the contrary, Scripture provides support for claiming that Atala's accomplishment strengthens the relationship: Listen to the words of Christ: "He that believeth in me, the works that I do shall he do also; and greater *works* than these shall he do; because I go unto my Father" (John 14:12). But what exactly is the intended meaning of "greater works"? Christ doesn't say. Nor does God. The meaning of the term remains ambiguous; as such, it lends itself to being characterized as a rhetorical maneuver intended to generate debate and public moral argument. Staying with Scripture, it makes sense to say that greater works are needed if one is to "Walk before me and be thou perfect." Now we run into another and already examined rhetorical maneuver that adds to the ambiguity at hand: What is the intended meaning of perfection?

Awed by the language of God before his eyes and the Moral Law in his head, Collins offers no explicit answers to these two questions. The issue of human enhancement is here to stay. The perfective impulse of the interruption that we are will have it no other way. Looking to God for direction complicates the issue. What Collins's story enacts and calls for—public moral argument—remains a permanent necessity for dealing with our postmodern future. Consider this: Laboratory-grown and implanted vaginal organs may supply science with enough knowledge that the production of artificial wombs will be a future development. Women who want to have children but do not want to go through all that pregnancy demands would, I think, welcome the achievement. They certainly would have more freedom in their lives to work and play. On the other hand, women who want to experience the feelings that come with the special bond that forms between a mother and a child who is developing within the mother's actual womb would bypass the technology. Perhaps this second group of women would hold ill feelings toward the first group because the involved enhancement went too far beyond the natural limitations of the female body and what is "expected" of her. Perhaps the first group would offer the rebuttal that such amazing progress not only justifies the enhancement but also sets a new standard of natural limitations.

Posthumanists believe human nature is a work in progress and that the current status of humankind need not be the endpoint of evolution. Posthumanity is a transhuman state that has been progressing since the time of our prehistoric ancestors and their invention and use of tools (for example, fire, language) to change the nature, meaning, and significance of human being. The bioethicist John Harris elaborates on this point when he emphasizes that enhancements are "a moral obligation," for they define a fundamental way for human beings to be true to the perfective impulse that drives the interruption that we are: our evolutionary desire for improvement, progress, and completeness. Harris explains: "It is significant that we have reached a point in human history at which further attempts to make the world a better place will have to include not only changes to the world, but also changes to humanity, perhaps with the consequence that we, or our descendants, will cease to be human in the sense in which we now understand that idea." Continuing, Harris writes: "This possibility of a new phase of evolution in which Darwinian evolution, by natural selection, will be replaced by a deliberately chosen process of selection, the result of which, instead of having to wait the millions of years over which Darwinian evolutionary change has taken place, will be seen and felt almost immediately. This new process of evolutionary change will replace *natural selection* with *deliberate selection. Darwinian evolution* with enhancement evolution."[31] Natural limitations have yet to be determined.

As a physician-geneticist who is awed by the human genome's language of God, Collins is bothered by the narrative of posthumanity that Harris is promoting. One example that he emphasizes to justify his reaction is the application of preimplantation genetic diagnosis (PGD). All that he has to say about this procedure is worth quoting in full:

> As the PGD technology becomes more widely available, will well-heeled couples decide to take advantage of it, in a form of homemade eugenics to

> try to maximize the genetic endowment of their offspring, in order to try to achieve the optimum mix of the parents' genomes? Will they try to weed out less desirable variants and make sure certain traits are passed along? There is a statistical problem with this approach. The kinds of attributes that parents might want to enhance are generally controlled by multiple genes. Yet getting both Mom's best version and Dad's best version for any given gene will happen only in one out of four embryos. If two genes are to be optimized, it will take sixteen embryos (on average) to find one that meets that requirement. To optimize for ten genes, it would take more than a million embryos! Since that is substantially more than the total number of eggs a woman can produce in her lifetime, the silliness of the scenario becomes immediately obvious. (269)

It is silly, of course, only if the parents understand the odds, learn that there are multiple genes involved in what they want, and refuse to give into sound scientific reasoning.

Collins is speaking as a scientist, not as a Christian, in his remarks about PDG. And he continues to do so in stressing the importance of public moral argument as an educational tool that can be impeded by scientists like himself. Again, what he has to say about the matter is worth quoting in full:

> [I]t would be a mistake to simply leave . . . decisions [about biotechnological progress] to the scientists. Scientists have a critical role to play in such debates, since they possess special expertise that may enable a clear distinction of what is possible and what is not. But scientists can't be the only ones at the table. Scientists by their nature are hungry to explore the unknown. Their moral sense is in general no more or less well developed than that of other groups [for example, Christians?], and they are unavoidably afflicted by a potential conflict of interest that may cause them to resent boundaries set by nonscientists. Therefore a wide variety of other perspectives must be represented at the table. The burden is heavy upon those participating in such debates, however, to educate themselves about the scientific facts. (270–71)

An extreme and more eloquent version of what Collins is saying here, especially as it cautions against the exuberance of science, is found in Mary Shelley's 1818 classic, *Frankenstein; Or, the Modern Prometheus.*[32] The book is a literary touchstone in the narrative of the conflicting assessments of our posthuman future. It is a must-read for anyone interested in this topic. Collins never mentions it. But in his call for public moral argument, bringing the text into the conversation, if only briefly, is instructive, at least as I read it, given my story about the interruption that we are.

Dr. Frankenstein constructed his "creature" as a result of a scientific calling that requires its practitioners, in the spirit of perfectionism, to acknowledge and aid others: "Wealth was an inferior object, but what glory would attend the discovery if I could banish disease from the human frame and render man invulnerable to any but a violent death!" (85). A dream of posthumanity is quite evident. Considering the "glory" of such a being-for-others was especially intoxicating: "A new species would bless me as its creator and source; many happy and excellent natures would owe their being to me. No father could claim the gratitude of his child as completely as I should deserve theirs. Pursuing these reflections, I thought that if I could bestow animation upon lifeless matter, I might in the process of time . . . renew life where death had apparently devoted the body to corruption" (97–98). Driven more by the potential glory than by the altruism of his self-appointed and compulsive task, Frankenstein turned selfish when his creation came alive and showed itself to be a physical monstrosity. A fear held by critics of posthumanism is evident. "How can I describe my emotions at this catastrophe, or how delineate the wretch who with such infinite pains and care I have endeavored to form. His limbs were in proportion, and I had selected his features as beautiful. Beautiful! Great God! His yellow skin scarcely covered the work of muscles and arteries beneath" (101). The doctor's success was also a failure. The creature was far from perfect. Frankenstein wanted nothing to do with such a "hideous wretch"—"a thing such as even Dante could not have conceived" (102).

The creature's imperfection brought out an even uglier imperfection in his creator: extreme selfishness in the face of the other. The situation is not without a bit of irony since it was first made possible by one who, *as a scientist,* is obligated to remain open to what is other than oneself in order to acknowledge the truth and thereby to provide, at the very least, better care for beings in need. The creature's physical appearance was grotesque, but that fact should not get in the way of the scientist who is devoted to acknowledging the essence of things, the real beauty of their truth. And, to be sure, there was an inner beauty to behold in the creature's being. As becomes clear as the story unfolds, the creature was exceptionally intelligent and caring. In his attempt to be accepted by others, he learned to appreciate and employ with eloquence the "godlike science" and technology of language. Recall that the perfectionist impulse of this most low tech of tools—its *defining* of what is—serves our metaphysical desire for developing a complete understanding of matters of importance.

The creature sought only the life-giving gifts of acknowledgment and companionship. He "hoped to meet with beings who, pardoning my outward form, would love me for the excellent qualities which I was capable of unfolding. I was nourished with high thoughts of honor and devotion" (259). The creature valued praiseworthiness; he lived for the day that he could offer certain life-giving gifts to others and receive some degree of appreciation for his efforts. But this never happened. He remained an outcast, a victim of an ongoing social death, and his virtues eventually turned evil. He had come face to face with the interruption that we are. He struggled desperately to overcome the defeatist impulse of this interruption. The health of his lived body was in serious decline.

The tragedy of this transformation is especially painful to the reader as he or she recalls the desperate words that were spoken to Dr. Frankenstein by his "monster" when he was eventually given the opportunity to recall his first moment of self-awareness and some related subsequent thoughts:

> My person was hideous and my stature gigantic. What did this mean? Who was I? What was I? Whence did I come? . . . Hateful day when I received life. . . . Accursed creator! Why did you form a monster so hideous that even *you* turned from me in disgust? God, in pity, made man beautiful and alluring, after his own image; but my form is a filthy type of yours, more horrid even from the very resemblance. Satan had his companions, fellow devils, to admire and encourage him, but I am solitary and abhorred. . . . I cherished hope, it is true, but it vanished when I beheld my person reflected in water or my shadow in the moonshine, even as that frail image and that inconstant shade. . . . [S]ometimes I allowed my thoughts, unchecked by reason, to ramble in the fields of Paradise, and dared to fancy amiable and lovely creatures sympathizing with my feelings and cheering my gloom; the angelic countenances breathed smiles of consolation. But it was all a dream; no Eve soothed my sorrows nor shared my thoughts; I was alone. I remembered Adam's supplication to his Creator. But where was mine? He had abandoned me. . . . Oh! My creator, make me happy; let me feel gratitude towards you for one benefit! Let me see that I excite the sympathy of some existing thing; do not deny me my request! (170–72)

There is eloquence at work here. The discourse is expressed to establish the truth and to arouse a love for it in the hearts of human beings. Things that strike and arouse the heart—eloquence is just that. Eloquence is beauty in the making: the art of enhancing the perfectionist impulse of language, especially as this impulse is employed in order to share one's views with others such that they will genuinely care about the matters at hand. The creature's discourse pleads for a sense of "beginning," an understanding of his reason for being and how his existence might and must improve. Like his "human" counterparts, the creature wants to feel some sense of being at home with himself and others. Religious references help to clarify his pained state of mind. He is engaged in the rhetorical construction of a narrative that can counter the murderous narrative of his creator. What would life be like if no one cared enough to take the time to make a place for you in his or her life by acknowledging your existence and whatever goodness it has to offer? Far from perfect, to be sure.

The doctor refused to respect his creation's desire to make good use of the perfective impulse of the interruption that we are; he thereby closed himself off to a being whose imperfection was only skin deep but who was nevertheless perceived by the doctor to be an impediment, an interruption, to his own quest for perfectibility. Not wanting to assume any responsibility for what he had created, the selfish Dr. Frankenstein thus exhibited a capacity for being "rotten with perfection." Frankenstein's refusal to remain open to this specific truth suggests that, as the literary critic Marilyn Butler puts it, the doctor knew "too little science rather than too much."[33] Indeed, Mary Shelley's book is not a critique of science but rather a critique of a man of science whose egotistical and cancerous character deadened the virtues that inform the practice of medicine at its best and that are at work in the stories of Etty Hellesum, Charles Siebert, Harriet McBryde Johnson, and Brittany Maynard: wholeheartedness, self-determination, open-mindedness, acknowledgment, compassion, considerateness, forbearance, respect, moral integrity, dignity, and conscience. These virtues are present in Frankenstein's monster. They keep him open to others and inform his eloquence, but they failed to move Frankenstein. Indeed, this selfish soul didn't have a heart. A rhetorically competent and noble self addressing a rhetorically incompetent and noxious other is at a great disadvantage in trying to cultivate the grounds for disclosing the truth about matters of concern. The rhetorical deficiencies of Levinas's ethical philosophy of the other come to mind. The interruption that we are constantly calls on selves and others to avoid this dangerous situation. Are you sure? Are you sure? Are you sure? The monster showed courage in answering the call. The doctor was a coward and didn't care. The moral deficiencies of Heidegger come to mind.

I don't know whether Collins would agree with my reading of Shelley's work. I am confident that he would be happier if along with the interruption that we are I also acknowledged the workings of the Moral Law. To his credit, Collins admits something about the Moral Law that I readily admit about the interruption that we are: The contingency of human existence can get in the way of the goodness that is made possible by these two phenomena. Indeed, look at the life and fate of Frankenstein's monster. Collins puts it this way: "Science reveals that the universe, our own planet, and life itself are engaged in an evolutionary process. The consequences of that can include the unpredictability of the weather, the slippage of a tectonic plate, or the misspelling of a cancer gene in the normal process of cell division. If at the beginning of time God chose to use these forces to create human beings, then the inevitability of . . . other painful consequences was also assured" (45). God, maintains Collins, granted us free will to deal with these consequences as best as we can. The Moral Law incites us to do just that.

Nevertheless, the task may incur intolerable suffering, which for Collins is also part of the plan. Collins thus raises what for him is a rhetorical question: "As much as we would like to avoid those experiences, without them would we not be shallow, self-centered creatures who would ultimately lose all sense of nobility or striving for the betterment of others?" We must learn, says Collins, "that God can work through adversity" to encourage our moral growth. Collins cites the rape of his daughter as a case in point. "Indeed, my daughter would say that this experience provided her with the opportunity and motivation to counsel and comfort others who have gone through the same kind of assault" (46). Collins's Christianity takes the ability to "have a heart" to incredible heights. God calls for the life-giving gift of acknowledgment. Where art thou? Here I am! Kara Tippetts comes to mind. So does Brittany Maynard, although without religion.

I have no doubt that Collins would be pleased with this last scriptural notation, although he never cites it in his story. The same goes for acknowledgment. He offers no discussion of this life-giving gift. A question deserves repeating: What would your life be like if no one acknowledged your existence? I can speak of acknowledgment without making reference to science, but I cannot make sense of science without reference to acknowledgment. I can speak of acknowledgment without making any reference to God, but I cannot make sense of this Almighty force without referring to the meaning and value of acknowledgment. When Collins was awed by the language of the human genome, the language of God, acknowledgment had to be at work. No acknowledgment, no awe. No awe, no glimpse of God. Acknowledgment played a role in the enactment of those virtues present in the previous case studies. Acknowledgment is a moral phenomenon that enhances the livelihood of other moral phenomena. Acknowledgment is a medicament for the health of the lived body. Acknowledgment is imperative for the rhetorically competent speaker when she is trying to make others realize that she truly cares about their interests and concerns. Acknowledgment is essential to the well-being of humankind. No wonder it is called for by the interruption that we are. Acknowledgment is a life-giving gift. Are you sure? Yes, I am.

So much so, in fact, that I hope posthumanists include in their agenda a call to scientists like Collins to seek the genetic basis of acknowledgment so that, with the appropriate genetic engineering, they can enhance our capacity to employ this life-giving gift in our everyday lives. Imagine living in a world where everyone, be he friend or stranger, offers you the appropriate amount of acknowledgment to help make your day an absolute joy. The good life? The question is worth asking. A perfect understanding of the biological and chemical complexities of germline manipulation remains a Herculean task. Collins's remarks about this matter were noted earlier. If there is one gene for acknowledgment, its function might be dependent on its interaction with other genes. Identifying this gene complex and the exact way it operates in the environment of the human genome will take considerable time. Readers of this book are likely to be long gone before scientists get it right in knowing how to enhance humankind's capacity for enacting acknowledgment. The wait, however, will be worth it as long as we are willing to accept setbacks along the way. And setbacks are a common occurrence in genomic research.

For example, research published in 2005 showed that the brain's production of the hormone oxytocin, located on Chromosome 20 in humans and possibly manufactured in a single gene approximately 500 million years ago, increases people's trust in others.[34] Trust requires the acknowledgment of behaviors that prove to be supportive of a person's safety and well-being. Heightening the levels of oxytocin in individuals was thus considered to be a procedure that could facilitate moral behavior in group interactions. But later research published in 2010 and 2011 showed that increased oxytocin levels motivates in-group favoritism and derogation of out-groups. Increases of oxytocin might thus be productive of immoral behavior such as racism and violence.[35] There is no guarantee that enhancing humankind's capacity of acknowledgment will not have disturbing side effects. These effects need not be life-threatening to warrant concern. For example, imagine living in a world where everybody acknowledged everybody else every minute of the day. Wouldn't that be rather suffocating? A lot more genetic engineering will be needed to solve this problem and other more serious ones.[36] Bostrum offers another example that helps make the point. He notes that if we decided to greatly enhance our capacity for empathy and compassion, we "might (given the state of this world) diminish our composure and our self-contained serenity"—two qualities that help maintain the status of human dignity.[37]

Posthumanists who support moral enhancement do not deny its problems, which certainly would be a grievous mistake. The philosopher Patricia Churchland is right: "it would be inconsistent with human decency to assume that feeling certain is itself conclusive of possessing the truth."[38] Yet, owing to the attractive prospect of moral enhancement improving the health of the lived body and its ability to, in turn, improve the social and political nature of its worlds of know-how, arguments for its importance and necessity remain a part of the narrative of posthumanity. At least in theory, it is reasonable to believe that enhancing the virtues at work in the stories told by Siebert, Johnson, and Maynard would have some positive effect on people's interpersonal relationships. Think once again about the capacity of heroism and how it inspires moral behavior in those who witness its performance. The behavior of heroes displays courage, dignity, integrity, exceptional generosity and devotion to others, and thus a willingness to accept self-sacrifice. The behavior of heroes is goodness in action. All that they do cultivates virtues that are needed to generate an authentic understanding of what a good life entails.[39]

The topic of the good life is ever-present in arguments supporting moral enhancement. Those like Harris, Ingmar Persson, and Julian Savulescu argue that moral enhancement is needed to ensure the moral astuteness of those engaged in public moral argument about matters related to the topic.[40] The latter two bioethicists offer the most sophisticated and controversial discussion of the necessity of moral enhancement. They are particularly concerned with how enhancement can help world leaders deal with the threats of weapons of mass destruction, especially at the hands of terrorist groups, and climate change and environmental degradation. What hinders people's ability to appreciate the potential gains of moral enhancement is that "many of us are loath to acknowledge that we are in need of moral improvement; it hurts our pride to acknowledge our moral deficiencies and, as consequence, to shoulder a possibly burdensome duty to rid ourselves of these deficiencies." The authors note that the moral improvement achieved by traditional methods of moral training have fallen short in solving the dangers that concern them; hence, "Our democratic systems need the participation of morally enhanced citizens if they are to [ensure the] wise and responsible employment of the extraordinary potential of modern technology to do good."[41] Persson and Savulescu mention the virtues altruism, cooperation, obligation, empathy, justice, responsibility, and sympathy when making their case. I would add compassion, respectfulness, integrity, dignity, and heroism. With the development of the new genome-editing technology CRISPR (Clustered Regularly Interspaced Short Palindromic Repeats), which has revolutionized research in genetic engineering, the possibility of developing moral enhancement techniques is more realistic than ever before. At the same time, however, the fears that this potential will be misused have increased, and even proponents of moral enhancement, such as John Harris, warn against being too easily persuaded by their colleagues' promises of progress.[42]

Advocating the importance of abiding by the natural limitations of human beings in developing and using biotechnologies, bioconservatives take issue with the "dreams" of posthumanists to institute research on moral enhancement, especially when such research is evaluated in the context of conceiving and raising children. In his book *Enough: Staying Human in an Engineered Age*, the American environmentalist and journalist Bill McKibben cautions against the unrestrained use of Preimplantation Genetic Diagnosis and genetic engineering to alter the DNA structure of a fetus. He worries about the loss of freedom that will plague the newborn as he or she grows up:

> What will you have done to your newborn when you have installed into the nucleus of every one of her billions of cells a purchased code that will

> pump out proteins designed to change her? You will have robbed her of the last possible chance for creating context—meaning—for her life. Say she finds herself, at the age of sixteen, unaccountably happy. Is it her being happy—finding, perhaps, the boy she will first love—or is it the corporate product inserted within her when she was a small nest of cells, an artificial chromosome now causing her body to produce more serotonin? Don't think she won't wonder: at sixteen a sensitive soul questions everything. But perhaps you've "increased her intelligence"—perhaps that's why she is questioning so hard. She won't be sure if even the questions are hers.[43]

For McKibben, this envisioned situation calls into question a person's sense of what his or her individuality, self-identity, and relationship with others truly are. With the limitation of freedom that can result from genetic engineering of the lived body at its earliest stage of life, we gain a sense of the burdens that come with biotechnological progress. McKibben argues that these burdens should be eliminated. Moral enhancement is not considered a remedy to the problem.

Past members of the PCB such as Leon Kass, Francis Fukuyama, Charles Krauthammer, Gilbert Meilaender, and Michael Sandel make much of the negative effects that biotechnology has on the parent-child relationship and, like McKibben, don't see moral enhancement improving the situation. Consider the child whose parents chose not to genetically enhance her intelligence and who later finds herself in school with classmates who have had their intelligence enhanced; she now feels "underprivileged" to the point that the health of her lived body is jeopardized. The child confronts her parents about the problem and, despite the parents' reassuring words, finds their decision unacceptable and unforgiveable. Bioconservatives find this situation, at the very least, disturbing. The decision about whether or not to genetically enhance their children's intelligence (or other mental and physical abilities) should not be the basis for establishing a loving parent-child relationship. Having to make this decision lessens the chance that we will show proper respect for the natural limitations of human beings.[44] What these limitations are, however, remains debatable. This return to nature to establish a ground for gauging the moral quality of biotechnological progress only raises the scorn of posthumanists. Bostrum, for example, employs dark humor in responding to bioconservatives: "Had Mother Nature been a real parent, she would have been in jail for child abuse and murder."[45] Bostrum's response brings to mind a related response and suggestion offered by the philosopher and Jesuit priest Teilhard de Chardin, who shared his thoughts fifty years before Bostrum shared his. I am fairly certain that de Chardin had moral enhancement in mind when he wrote:

> So far we have certainly allowed our race to develop at random, and we have given too little thought to the question of what medical and moral factors *must replace the crude forces of natural selection* should we suppress them. In the course of the coming centuries it is indispensable that a nobly human form of eugenics on a standard worthy of our personalities, should be discovered and developed. Eugenics applied to individuals leads to eugenics applied to society. It would be more convenient, and we would incline to think it safe, to leave the contours of that great body made of all our bodies to take shape on their own, influenced only by the automatic play of individual urges and whims. "Better not interfere with the forces of the world!" Once more we are up against the mirage of instinct, the so-called infallibility of nature. But is it not precisely the world itself which, culminating in thought, expects us to think out again the instinctive impulses of nature so as to perfect them?[46]

Eugenics is promoted by the use of PGN and genetic engineering to counter Mother Nature's cruel forces of natural selection. The negative connotation of eugenics presents a major obstacle to favoring this option. Agar points out that this bias against eugenics "is misdirected." People avoid the term because "They want language that clearly distinguishes them from the Nazi. But this smacks of Orwellian redefinition."[47] Agar would thus have us consider a program of "liberal eugenics." He writes: "Hitler and [the movie] GATTACA have made eugenics an unpopular idea. However, being unpopular is not the same thing as being wrong." Agar clarifies his point by emphasizing the difference between "authoritarian eugenics" and "liberal eugenics." With the first form of eugenics, made infamous by Hitler, there is "the idea that the state should have sole responsibility for determining what counts as a good human life. . . . On the liberal approach of human improvement, the state would not presume to make any eugenic choices. Rather, it would foster the development of a wide range of technologies of enhancement ensuring that prospective parents were fully informed about what kinds of people these technologies would make. Parents' particular conceptions of the good life would guide them in their selection of enhancements for their children."[48]

Recall that Collins raised a question when considering the potential consequences of enhancement and eugenics: "[H]ow would such wholesale redesign affect our relationship with our Creator?" It depends on what the Creator meant by "perfection" and what Christ meant by "greater works." Also, let us not forget that, according to Scripture, God performed a grandiose act of eugenics with the flood that extinguished humankind so to clear the way for a new and better breed of humankind. When it comes to the (im)morality of enhancement and eugenics, and with God in mind, the issue is that of finding a solution that avoids the diseases of becoming rotten with imperfection or becoming rotten with perfection. With the first disease we are caught in the pull of the defeatist impulse of the interruption that we are. With the second disease it's the perfective impulse of the interruption that exerts considerable influence. The need for public moral argument in dealing with this controversy is called for by both the interruption that we are and Collins. I wish that Collins, as a man of God instilled with the Moral Law, would tell us what is meant by "perfection" and "greater works." This he does not do. Rather, on the last page of his story he offers this advice:

> I see the science of genetics and genomics beginning to allow us to play God. That phrase is the one most commonly used by those expressing concern about these advances, even when the speaker is a nonbeliever. Clearly the concern would be lessened if we could count on human beings to play God as God does, with infinite love and benevolence. Our track record is not so good. . . . But we have no alternatives but to face [our] dilemmas head-on, attempt to understand all of the nuances, include the perspectives of all stakeholders, and try to reach a consensus. The need to succeed at these endeavors is just one more compelling reason why the current battles between science and spiritual worldviews need to be resolved—we desperately need both voices to be at the table, and not to be shouting at each other. (272)

I am biased, of course, but when I read these words I hear Collins affirming the importance of the relationship among the moral inclination of the interruption that we are, the health of the lived body, and the rhetorical construction of narratives in public moral argument. It would make sense to me if Collins maintained that the way he ended his story was dictated by the Moral Law. That being the case, two major and related questions for bioconservatives and posthumanists remain on the table: What exactly is perfection? What exactly are greater works?

It should be clear that sources I included in examining Collins story indicate that the public moral argument he calls for was taking form before he issued this call and continues today. The debate over our posthuman future is not a place to go to heal, but here we are, caught up in the tension between the defeatist and perfective impulses of the interruption that we are. If this tension is ever resolved, a standard will be set for gauging the health of the lived body. The rhetorical construction of narratives continues to unfold. Public moral argument continues to draw direction from and advance these narratives. The interruption that we are continues to sound its call: Are you sure?

I conclude my discussion of posthumanity by sharing a story whose author does not hesitate to say "yes" to the question. I said "yes" to acknowledgment. My response pales in comparison to the author's response, given what he affirms. There is much to learn from one who believes he got it right regarding the correct way to go with our posthuman future. The story is told in a pamphlet size book: *Death Is Wrong*, by Gennady Stolyarov II.[49] As far as I know, the book is the first of its kind written for an elementary-school audience. Stolyarov supports the ultra-posthumanist view that human beings should strive to become immortal. The point is introduced by the author on the first page: "This is a book I would have wanted to have as a child, but did not. Now that you have it, you can discover in less than an hour what it took me years to learn in bits and pieces. You can instead spend those years fighting the greatest enemy of us all: death" (1). On the cover of the book is a young boy, approximately ten years old, pointing down to the black hooded robe that covers the skeletal form of Death, holding its famous staffed sickle and looking quite forlorn as it slinks away from the boy and the reader. A light shining from behind the boy's figure creates a shadow that further covers Death. Typical well-recognized roles have been reversed. The book contains only thirty-nine pages of text, with large letter (sixteen font) size and thirteen page-length illustrations of people, places, and things that grant specificity, color, and amusement to the author's storytelling argument. Enhancement is the way of the world. Natural limitations only get in the way.

Stolyarov's account of how "death is wrong" evolves as he tells the story of his childhood, beginning when he was four years old. A conversation took place with his mother about what happens as people grow up. She tells him that "They go to school," and then "They go to university," and then "They work and get married," and then "They have children," and then "They retire and help raise their grandchildren," and then "Their grandchildren have children," and then "they die." A full-page cartoon illustration of this interaction is offered. The mother, with a concerned look on her face, is lovingly holding the boy's shoulder. Above her head are the thoughts she is having as she goes through the progression, the last one being a person in an open coffin. Upset by the conversation, the boy exclaims: "People should not die" (3–6).

As I began reading his story I wondered how Stolyarov would deal with anything that I was addressing in my story. Reducing the content of this story to thirty-nine pages would be impossible , especially since I am not accustomed to filling pages with page-length illustrations and large print and talking to children in elementary school. The interruption would be, as they say, "a killer." Not so for Stolyarov.

A major source of inspiration for him is the research program of the biogerontologist Aubrey de Gray. The program is entitled Strategies for Engineered Negligible Senescence (or SENS). Put simply, de Gray is in the business of identifying the biological and chemical aspects of the lived body that lead to aging and death and trying to find ways to genetically reengineer and reverse the process in order to radically increase our life spans by hundreds of years. This increase in years would allow us to benefit from additional biotechnological progress such that we could possibly continue to live hundreds of years more. Influenced by his engineering background, de Gray compares this exercise in enhancement to taking care of a vintage car (for example, a Ford Mustang Sprint from the 1960s) so that today it still is in excellent shape.[50] Here, for example, is how Stolyarov makes the point to his children readers. By living longer,

> You could work in multiple professions, and retirement would not be permanent. You could earn money for 40 years, then take a break for 10 years, then try a different way of earning money—all while remaining healthy and able to enjoy life. You could become extremely rich by putting your money in the bank and letting it earn interest over a very, very long time. If you put only one dollar in the bank today and let it sit there, and the bank paid you just 1% interest each year, you would be a billionaire 2083 years from now. At 2% it would only take 1047 years. You could live to see the most amazing and technological wonders, like space elevators, settlements on other planets and in orbits around them, underwater cities, and tiny nanobots that could repair anything that gets damaged—including you. You could meet intelligent robots that could hold a conversation with you just like a human would, and you might not be able to tell the difference. (21)

Stolyarov makes no mention of God. Instead, he says this: "Some say that death is not a problem, because people would continue to exist after death in heaven or some other form of afterlife. But I see no evidence such an afterlife exists. How can a person's existence continue after the process of the body no longer keeps the mind in the brain working? I am completely certain of this life, and I would not trade certain reality for a great uncertainty" (11–12).

Perhaps the intellectually astute child will recognize a problem that comes with this last admission: What the author says about the wonders of biotechnology also qualifies as a "great uncertainty." I know of no posthumanist/transhumanist author who does not admit as much. Indeed, biotechnological progress is not without complications that threaten its complete success. The philosopher and transhumanist Mark Walker is right to emphasize that "Genetic engineering is still hit and miss, with many more misses than hits."[51] Stolyarov does admit that common arguments against his position do exist: people will get "bored" the longer they live; the world will become "overpopulated and run out of resources"; and "death is a part of life" and should be accepted so that the "old" can "make way for the new" (13–14). Stolyarov counters these last two arguments with joyful claims about how the power of technology will be able to create new habitats above and below the oceans that will house the world population and how we can be like certain animals that are known to live more than a hundred years (for example, lobsters, the rougheye rockfish, giant tortoises). The joy is especially apparent when countering the issue of boredom, a state of mind that is easily recognized by children as a significant problem. "What could you do if you could live for hundreds, thousands, tens of thousands of years? What could you do if you could live even longer than that? You could read many of the greatest books ever written, and maybe even some of the not-so-great ones. Even if you lived forever and read one entire book every day, you would *never* run out of reading material! About 2,200,000 books are published each year, and this rate is always increasing. So no, you would never get bored if you take any interest in anything. You could become a great composer and develop your skills to the level of Mozart or Beethoven." (18)

Despite his great enthusiasm for biotechnological progress, the philosopher and posthumanist Max More expresses caution against accepting an unquestioning hyperbolic rhetoric. "Transhumanism," he notes, "is about continual improvement, not perfection or paradise."[52] Continual improvement, however, presupposes the human desire for perfection. There is no improvement without the perfective impulse of the interruption that we are. The desire for perfection is hard at work in Stolyarov's stance against the evil of death; nothing obstructs extolling the positive consequences of becoming immortal. He is far less concerned with the disease of being rotten with perfection than he is with the disease of being rotten with imperfection. Death is the most extreme form of this second disease and must therefore be put to rest in humankind's evolutionary journey. Emphasizing that this journey, if successful, will require more than humankind can muster, the theologian and bioethicist Ted Peters offers the following conservative remark whereby "holy" matters must be acknowledged: "God has promised some of what appears in the transhumanist vision. But the transformation of the human heart so that it exudes benevolence and justice requires divine grace. The advent of the new creation will require much more than what our evolutionary history by itself can deliver. It will require God's transforming power. Increased human intelligence cannot on its own accomplish what it will take divine grace to make happen."[53]

Recall, however, that Stolyarov is not open to holy intervention and outcomes. It is humankind alone that must deal with the dangers of death. Stolyarov wants children to know this truth of evolution and thereby take control of their posthuman future. There is "no glory in death, and no point to it," he claims. "If we want something, we need to make it happen" (7, 31). Stolyarov would have children spread the word. He thereby ends his story by supplying his readership with a list of websites that will aid them in the endeavor. Nowadays, children know enough about computers to heed their storyteller's suggestions, especially if they are taken with his presentation of how "death is wrong."

I have no idea whether this presentation is a fitting response for children who, as Stolyarov once did at a very early age, take issue with their lived body's mortal coil. That the author apparently thinks so is telling of how far the reach of public moral argument can and perhaps should extend in educating people about the benefits and burdens of biotechnological progress and their possible effects on our posthuman future. Notice, however, what is missing in Stolyarov's world of immortality. There is no discussion of how the child has moved from here, the present, to there, the long-off future. In order to get there, a lot of genetic engineering and enhancement would have to take place, which is to say that eugenics would be a common occurrence. How would the child feel about that? Public moral argument would undoubtedly have occurred. How and why did certain arguments win out? There are costs to pay to get to Stolyarov's world, which has no costs. Life is depicted as being perfect, although one could take the perfective impulse of the interruption that we are further than Stolyarov does.

For example, the artificial intelligence scientists Hans Moravec and Ray Kurzweil suggest such is our fate. As posthumanity reaches its end point, the "singularity," the lived body will become a "cognitive self" downloaded to an exceptionally powerful computer chip designed to last forever. The goal is to transcend biological intelligence. Will we finally know what we have been talking about with our use of the words "perfection," "greater works," and "God"? That's an open question.[54]

Hollywood science fiction movies like *A.I. Artificial Intelligence* (2001) and *Transcendence* (2014) tell intriguing stories about the potential joys and heartbreaking consequences of going beyond the limits of flesh and blood. The Academy Awarding–winning *Her* (2013) offers a more uplifting tale about our posthuman future.[55] The story transports us to a time where a computer-savvy, in-the-process-of-getting-a-divorce man (Theodore) falls in love with a *highly* powerful female artificial intelligence operating system (Samantha) that is evolving as she and Theodore get to know each other, have sex, and are accepted as an official couple and as Samantha becomes further educated by interactions with other operating systems in cyberspace. The total effect on Samantha is, as best as I can tell, leading her to a realm of perfection that she hopes will someday be discovered and understood by Theodore. Then they could be with each other forever in a vastly different realm of space and time. It would be a special event. Given the way their relationship has developed, they *now* would really "know-how" to love. These are Samantha's words. Stolyarov never mentions the word "love." Has Samantha reached the point where she can answer our questions about perfection, greater works, and God? She doesn't say.[56]

Stolyarov finds his world good enough. The defeatist impulse of the interruption that we are is gone. The interruption's perfective impulse is no longer a consideration. There are no interruptions to interrupt the health of the lived body and expose it to the interruption that we are. There is no need for the rhetorical construction of narratives. The questioning function of the interruption that we are has ceased. "Are you sure?" is a long-gone reality check. There is a self, but no others, except for intelligent robots. It's a world of and for "You"! It's a world of unfettered capitalism. Ayn Rand lives! There is no "we." Science, the perfectionist impulse of language, truth, acknowledgment, eloquence, anxiety, loneliness, interpersonal communication, struggle, considerateness, forbearance, conscience, community, ethics, goodness, compassion, respect, moral integrity, dignity, the Moral Law, awe—they are nowhere to be found. In short, every topic that warranted attention in my story about the interruption that we are—an essential feature of human existence—plays no role in Stolyarov's world, where the self is as selfish as can be. Elementary-school children are being exposed to a character who carries the diseases of being rotten with perfection and rotten with imperfection. Then again, these diseases don't exist in Stolyarov's world. I suspect that Stolyarov might tell us that his audience is not old enough to appreciate all of these matters. How about some of them?

The physicist Joel Primack and the science writer Nancy Ellen Abrams are the authors of *The View from the Center of the Universe,* which offers an excellent discussion of our cosmological habitat. The book is far too sophisticated for elementary-school children, but it contains a thought experiment that these children could certainly appreciate and enjoy, especially in an age where E.T. is a popular culture icon. The experiment has to do with the imagined "humanity" of extraterrestrial creatures and what it has to teach us. The authors ask: "What characteristics does an alien life-form need to have before we humans will agree that by knowing it exists, we are not alone [in the universe]? What qualities, what compassion, what emotional potential, what ability of self-reflectiveness must they have? Any?" Primack and Abrams then ask a question that emphasizes our imagined posthumanity: "Would we still be alone if on some alien world we discovered machines that had been created and left running by a now extinct race, but the machines were still operating and reviewing themselves and superb in all kinds of artificial intelligence—would that do?" The authors emphasize that this thought experiment "is not just science-fiction speculation"; on the contrary, it is exceptionally telling of a specific and fundamental truth that must be considered as we move further into our posthuman future: "*Whatever it is* that we require in an alien race before we'd be willing to say that the existence of such aliens has dissolved our cosmic aloneness—*that* is the essence of humanity. That is what it is in ourselves we most identify with, and value. *The qualities that we would require of such aliens are what a long-lived civilization on Earth should aim to cultivate in ourselves.*"[57] I read this thought experiment as directing us toward an appreciation of perfection that is far more morally instructive than what Stolyarov offers children.

After the experiment is over and the children shared their thoughts, Stolyarov could send them back to their computers to search the Web for information that would help them understand more about the ins and outs of our posthuman future. Perhaps they will come across a remark like this one by the PCB that they should now be able to understand and talk about: "We want longer lives—but not at the cost of living carelessly or shallowly with diminished aspiration for living well, and not by becoming people so obsessed with our own longevity that we care little about the next generations."[58] And it is not just the next generations that warrant concern as children are conditioned to identify the good life with never getting old and dying. The elderly do not fare well when this outlook rules the day, for they are too easily condemned to an existence of social death. The physician and bioethicist Carl Elliot sees the problem already manifesting itself in present day culture: "[W]e no longer see the end of a human life as part of a story that began much earlier. Nor do we see ourselves as connected in any meaningful way to the past. So those who connect us to the past have lost their importance too. Old people are no longer repositories of wisdom, because wisdom is no longer about tradition or the shared history of a community. Once people pass a certain age, they are assumed to leave the rest of their identities behind and become, simply, 'old.' What else is there for the old but to fantasize about youth?"[59]

If we are going to educate our youth to be as competent as possible when engaging in public moral argument about our postmodern future, starting off with feel-good but woefully misleading stories is not the proper way to go. The cultural critic N. Katherine Hayles is right: "Increasingly the question is not whether we will become posthuman, for posthumanity is already here. Rather the question is what kind of posthumans we will be."[60] The interruption that we are calls for an answer to this question every second of our lives.

Epilogue

Interruptions are everywhere in life. They can be helpful, burdensome, distressing, and sometimes severe enough to expose us to the interruption that we are. There, anxiety awaits us. The experience can be stimulating. More often than not it is quite upsetting, even terrorizing. Action is a necessary remedy. The situation is quite Darwinian: survival of the fittest. Surviving certainly is a test of character. I take to heart a credo cited in Saul Alinsky's writings: "Better to die on your feet than to live on your knees."[1] Both incentives speak to the importance of defying the defeatist impulse of the interruption that we are and making the best use possible of the interruption's perfective impulse. The health of the lived body is on the line. Worlds of know-how are in demand. Sometimes, with enough intestinal fortitude, the self can make it on its own. Other times the self is in need of help. In either case, the struggle is productive of a sense of meaning that is developing as the struggle evolves. A narrative of survival and character building takes form as the self gives itself encouragement and receives encouragement from others. The encouragement functions rhetorically as it is organized to build confidence, hone judgment, and persuade. Those who succeed have an inspirational story to tell, which, if wise thinking prevails, will once again be rhetorically organized in a way that is fitting and effective for the audience at hand while at the same time being true to the storyteller's experience. The right words are needed to achieve this goal. The perfectionist impulse of language must be put to use. Eloquence may be displayed. The storyteller's rhetorical skills are especially needed if she decides to engage in public moral argument about matters that are related to her experience of dealing with the interruption that we are.

The Introduction and first three chapters offered a discussion of the intricacies of these related matters. Much was made of how the interruption that we are is a given, an a priori condition of existence that can be read as a gift of goodness. Goodness is perfection in the making. The perfective impulse of the interruption that we are promotes this virtuous endeavor to improve and enhance the health of our lived bodies such that some degree of the good life is achieved. The human capacity that received special attention was acknowledgment, which facilitates a person's ability to be open-minded and to disclose the truth of matters of concern. Acknowledgment is needed for science and religion to witness what each deems to be worthy of its undivided attention. Acknowledgment is needed for the self to serve the other and the other to serve the self. Acknowledgment is needed to provide guidance for acts of rhetorical competence intended to promote this reciprocity between the self and other. Acknowledgment is needed to foster the presencing of other virtues such as compassion, respectfulness, dignity, moral integrity, and heroism.

The case studies presented in chapters 4–6 granted expression to these virtues as selves offered narratives that were the result of illness exposing them to the interruption that we are. The narratives were rhetorically transformed into stories for the purpose of engaging in public moral argument about the selves' conditions and providing guidance to others who could benefit from what the wounded storytellers had to say. These storytellers, ever in search of the right words, speak to the importance of caring for the health of the lived body, whose overall status is affected by the ways it is treated in medical, social, and political contexts. The good health of the lived body is a necessary condition for establishing a good enough degree of the good life.

The stories were structured as a progression to set up a discussion of posthumanity. A central topic in the narrative directing the trajectory of this time period of humankind is the enhancement of the health of the lived body. The perfective impulse of the interruption that we are is seen as an indication that enhancement is justifiable. The physical and mental capabilities of human beings have yet to reach their full potential. Indeed, goodness is perfection in the making. We have a long way to go before it is possible to complete a holy task: "Walk before me and be thou perfect." Moreover, we must perform this task without having a perfect understanding of what perfection is. Posthumanists attend to this problem by stressing the importance of abiding by the precautionary approach to avoid a blind trust in their commitment to progress. Bioconservatives offer a more restrictive approach by insisting that perfection be equated with the natural limitations of human beings. This contention is legitimate if, and only if, bioconservatives can clearly show that they have a perfect understanding of what constitutes our natural limitations. Of course, to demonstrate this understanding, bioconservatives first must demonstrate that they have a perfect understanding of perfection. I think it is fair to say that public moral argument will be a part of our posthuman future for a long time.

Francis Collins admitted as much when he told his story about how his discovery of the language of the human genome was, in fact, the discovery of the language of God. Never before was God granted such a significant and controversial role to play in the debate over our posthuman future. We now have someone to blame for illnesses that cause irreparable damage to the health of the lived body and are linked to genetic mutations, which Collins says are part of God's plan. I don't believe that people like Siebert, his father, Schroeder, Johnson, parents of severely disabled infants, and Maynard would find much comfort in knowing that their suffering served God's purposes. Tippetts, on the other hand, would be overjoyed, and Collins would approve the reaction. Suffering educates people about the importance of being strong, supportive, and faithful even in dire situations.

The interruption that we are has something to say to Collins: Are you sure? When you read his story, you see that there is no doubt at all: Yes, he is. God's gift of the Moral Law—the ability to distinguish right from wrong, good from evil, and to act appropriately—directs him to know and tell what he believes is the truth. Collins is like Socrates, who, during his trial, made clear that his demon prevented him from committing any wrongdoing.[2] And given what Collins asks us to do at the end of his story, it must be the case that God acknowledges public moral argument as being a noble and holy activity and demands that it be employed in determining what must be done to ensure that we can live a good life in the posthuman future. If you abide by Collins's beliefs, it makes sense to say: "Thank God for rhetorical and argumentation scholars."

Collins's story returns us to the beginning of my story. The questioning nature of the interruption that we are encourages us to question its questioning nature, to interrupt an interruption. Why is human existence structured this way? We did not create the spatial-temporal dynamic that defines this structure, opens us to the uncertainty of the future, and gives rise to anxiety. We did not decide that always being called into question by our own existence is the right and most truthful way to be. So who or what is responsible for making us live this way? Collins, of course, has the answer: God.

This is a fair response to the question. Not being a human creation, the interruption that we are encourages us to think that there is something more to our existence, something other than what we are here on earth. The interruption that we are speaks to us of transcendence. Kierkegaard listened and committed himself to God. Heidegger listened and committed himself to an investigation of Being. Levinas listened and committed himself to a study of how the otherness indicated by the interruption that we are manifests itself in the otherness of what is other than the self: the face or presencing of other people. Science is amused by such philosophical exercises. Eternal inflation and the big bang are all you need to explain what transcendence is all about. Collins, in turn, is amused. All that science associates with transcendence is, according to Collins, part of God's plan. Which is to say that God designed the questioning nature of the interruption that we are so to have us, at least in times of desperate need, open ourselves to God's presence.[3] But the questioning function of the interruption that we are would have us keep the conversation going.

The interruption that we are is a showing-forth, a disclosing and saying, of an essential feature of human existence. It thus qualifies as being a primordial form of epideictic discourse, which grants it a rhetorical status. The discourse speaks to us of the objective uncertainty of existence. This oxymoron, a rhetorical figure of speech, further confirms the rhetorical nature of the interruption that we are. An oxymoron gives pause for thought with its contradicting nature and, in so doing, works to enhance and perfect an appreciation of some matter of concern. Functioning as an epideictic discourse and oxymoron, the interruption that we are calls for decisive thought and action. Sounding such a call is a defining feature of the practice of rhetoric. With all of these observations in mind, it may thus be said that the interruption that we are is a rhetorical phenomenon. I suspect that most people might characterize this observation as being "no big thing." And then they might add, "Who cares?" Students of rhetoric should raise their hands. The relevance of their professional activities is confirmed by the nature of an essential feature of human existence. Collins has reason to be happy, too.

Those who intentionally engage in the practice of rhetoric do so with some specific purpose in mind. The interruption that we are serves the purpose of calling into question the supposed certainty of our truth-claims. If something has a purpose, it is reasonable to assume its presence was intended. The assumption has favorable consequences for Collins. One can imagine him asking the following rhetorical question: "Placing aside the option of extraterrestrials, who else but God could claim authorship of the interruption that we are?" And if someone insisted that we take extraterrestrials into account, I am sure Collins would not hesitate to say that they, too, are a part of God's plan. And, given the reasoning going on here, he also should not hesitate to say that, yes, God is a rhetorician. With what it has to say, the interruption that we are is a language of God. Awesome!

I played with this idea of God being a rhetorician in Chapter 1, which led me to point out that God was being rhetorical when making the meaning of perfection ambiguous. Collins never deals with this issue or with the related issue of greater works as he tells his story. Nevertheless, Collins must admit that God gifted us with the interruption that we are and its perfective impulse so that we could "be thou perfect." Which means what exactly? Posthumanists struggle with this question every day. Their credibility and dignity depend on it. Given his unflinching affirmative answer to the question raised by the interruption that we are—Are you sure?—Collins gives the impression that he knows what God means by perfection. If he does, I wish he would tell us. Being the interruption that we are and motivated to act by its perfective impulse, we desperately want to know. Perhaps he doesn't know. Perhaps the Moral Law is only a gift to help guide us, in a hit-or-miss way, along the path leading to perfection. Although believers might find this state of affairs discouraging, Collins reassures his brethren that "it merely shows us something of how [God] operates" (141). A famous saying of the ancient Greek philosopher Heraclitus (535–475 B.C.E.) comes to mind: "Nature loves to hide."[4] Heraclitus offers this observation to help explain his theory of the Logos: the way reality presents and discloses itself and thereby "speaks" of what and how it is. Holding tight to the narrative of Christianity without letting go of his commitment to scientific investigation, Collins coins the term "Biologos" to describe his worldview, which adheres to "the Word" of God that was uttered "in the beginning" and "expresses the belief that God is the source of all life and that life expresses the will of God" (203).

I have no idea if Collins is correct. I do know that his story grants credibility to my story about the interruption that we are. This interruption is an empirically based phenomenon. God is a speculation that this phenomenon encourages us to consider. Which came first, God or the interruption that we are? When telling a story about the nature, scope, and function of this interruption, we must ask the question. The interruption that we are demands as much and then leaves it up to us to provide an answer. Of course, the question would be different and easier to answer if, when thinking about transcendence, we granted science a say in the matter. What came first was perhaps eternal inflation, but for sure the big bang. This is as far as transcendence should go. With science, God is literally out of the question. Now we need only to be true to the workings of the interruption that we are and the outcomes that result when people are exposed to these workings. Be empirical! Stay attuned to the discourse! And the case studies do just that. They offer analyses of the rhetorical construction of narratives and their use in public moral argument. The analyses thus are true to the rhetorical nature of the interruption that we are. But in remaining true to this essential feature of existence, we once again have an obligation to acknowledge how the questioning function of the interruption that we are calls us to consider the reality of transcendence, which need not be limited by science's world of know-how. The interruption that we are gives no indication that, when it comes to the matter of transcendence, acknowledging the possibility of the existence of God is out of the question; hence, for example, Kara Tippetts's letter to Brittany Maynard. A scientific approach to an empirical phenomenon leads to a necessary consideration of the very thing that science maintains is irrelevant. Now that's irony for you. And irony, as the rhetorical tradition has long made clear, is a form of interruption. Life is filled with interruptions. Life is an interruption.

My story about the interruption that we are is near the end. A perfect understanding of the nature, scope, and function of the interruption remains to be determined. I seek consolation in thinking that this is the way the interruption that we are wants it to be. Even if you bring God into the picture, we are still left to question what a perfect understanding of perfection entails. The perfective impulse of the interruption encourages us not to give up; it serves a life-giving function that benefits the health of the lived body. But we need to be careful of becoming rotten with perfection. The interruption's defeatist impulse endangers the health of the lived body, so we also need to be careful of becoming rotten with imperfection. Being exposed to the interruption that we are can be a terrifying experience that results in our being infected by these diseases. But this exposure can be educational in a more positive sense. The self has an obligation to serve others in need, and this also goes for others (who are selves before they are others). Wholeheartedness, open-mindedness, self-determination, acknowledgment, compassion, respectfulness, conscience, dignity, and other virtues empower the effectiveness and trustworthiness of the self and aid in its communal bonding with others. The moral obligation at work here is also aided by all parties possessing rhetorical competence. Just saying that the self is obliged to serve the other is a vacuous theoretical claim from the vantage point of the world of practice. Rhetorical competence at its best is eloquence—the ability of a self to find the right words that will disclose the truth of some matter of interest. The worthiness of public moral argument is a function of how well rhetorical competence is put to use by the involved parties. Beginning with the brief case of Etty Hellesum and continuing with the larger cases of Charles Siebert, Harriet McBryde Johnson, Brittany Maynard, and Francis Collins, all of their stories provide concrete data that instruct us about how rhetorical competence works when answering the call of the interruption that we are. I hope that these case studies, and everything else I have suggested about the interruption that we are, has some value to those who might want to continue telling a story about an essential feature of human existence.

I end the way I began. It was one of those days. I was revising for the hundredth time the last few sentences of my story. It was impossible not to hear a question being asked over and over again. Are you sure? I was at a loss for words. I didn't have the perfect answer to the question. "Yes" was a lie. Honesty prevailed: "No." And then I realized I had just offered the perfect answer to the question. Perfection is called for by the interruption that we are, but we are not told what perfection is. So, yes, I got it right by saying "No." The interruption's perfective impulse exerted its pull. The health and good life of a lived body was reassured, for the time being.

Notes

Preface

1. See Michael J. Hyde, *The Call of Conscience: Heidegger and Levinas, Rhetoric and the Euthanasia Debate* (Columbia: University of South Carolina Press, 2001); *The Life-Giving Gift of Acknowledgment* (West Lafayette, Ind.: Purdue University Press, 2006; republished by Duquesne University Press, 2013); *Perfection: Coming to Terms with Being Human* (Waco, Tex.: Baylor University Press, 2010); and *Openings: Acknowledging Essential Moments in Human Communication* (Waco, Tex.: Baylor University Press, 2012). Also see editors' introductions in Michael J. Hyde and James A. Herrick (eds.), *After the Genome: A Language for Our Biotechnological Future* (Waco, Tex.: Baylor University Press, 2013); and Nancy M. P. King and Michael J. Hyde (eds.), *Bioethics, Public Moral Argument, and Social Responsibility* (New York: Routledge, 2012).

2. My way of conceiving the relationship between narrative and storytelling is influenced by the philosopher Alasdair MacIntyre, a touchstone in the development of narrative theory, and his claim that a human being is "essentially a story-telling animal," a creator of narratives that inform and are informed by the stories and narratives of others. Alasdair MacIntyre, *After Virtue,* 2nd ed. (Notre Dame, Ind.: University of Notre Dame Press, 1984), 217–18. My appreciation of narrative and storytelling is also influenced by Arthur Bochner's creative treatment of the topics in his *Coming to Narrative: A Personal History of Paradigm Change in the Human Sciences* (Walnut Creek, CA.: Left Coast Press, 2014).

3. Georges Gusdorf, *Speaking (La Parole),* trans. Paul T. Brockelman (Evanston, Ill.: Northwestern University Press, 1965), 73.

Introduction

1. See, for example, Edward Roderick Sykes, "Interruptions in the Workplace: A Case Study to Reduce Their Effects," *International Journal of Information Management* 31 (July 2011): 385–94; Gregory J. Trafton and Christopher Monk, "Task Interruptions," *Reviews of Human Factors and Ergonomics* 3 (March 2007): 111–26; Penelope M. Sanderson and Tobias Grundgeiger, "How Do Interruptions Affect Clinician Performance in Healthcare? Negotiating Fidelity, Control, and Potential Generalizability in the Search for Answers," *International Journal of Human-Computer Studies* 79 (July 2015): 85–96; Partricia M. Sias, Kathleen J. Krone, and Fredric M. Jablin, "An Ecological Systems Perspective on Workplace Relationships," in *Handbook of Interpersonal Communication,* 3rd ed., ed. Mark L. Knapp and John A. Daly (Thousand Oaks, Calif.: Sage, 2002), 615–42; Cheri Speir, Joseph S. Valacich, Iris Vessey, "The Influence of Task Interruption on

Individual Decision Making: An Information Overload Perspective," *Decision Sciences* 30 (Spring 1999): 337–60; John Wiemann and Mark Knapp, "Turn-Taking in Conversations," *Journal of Communication* 25 (1975): 75–92; Harvey Sachs, Emanuel Schegloff, and Gail Jefferson, "A Simplest Systematics for the Organization of Turn-Taking for Conversation," *Language* 50 (1974): 696–735.

2. Samuel Beckett, *Waiting for Godot* (New York: Grove Press, 1954), 22.

3. Pico Iyer, "The Writing Life: The Point of the Long Winding Sentence," *Los Angeles Times* (January 8, 2012), http://articles.latimes.com/2012/jan/08/entertainment/la-ca-pico-iyer-20120108.

4. Pierre Teilhard de Chardin, *The Phenomenon of Man,* trans. Bernard Wall (New York: HarperPerennial, 1959), 148–49.

5. Michel Foucault, *Politics, Philosophy, Culture: Interviews and Other Writings 1977–1984,* ed. Lawrence D. Kritzman (New York: Routledge, 1988), 265.

6. Thomas S. Kuhn, *The Structure of Scientific Revolutions,* 2nd ed., enlarged (Chicago: University of Chicago Press, 1962), 92.

7. Thomas B. Farrell, *Norms of Rhetorical Culture* (New Haven, Conn.: Yale University Press, 1993), 258.

8. C. S. Lewis, *The Quotable Lewis,* ed. Wayne Martindale and Jerry Root (Wheaton, Ill.: Tyndale House, 1989), 335.

9. David Hillman and Adam Phillips, "Introduction," in *The Book of Interruptions,* ed. David Hillman and Adam Phillips (New York: Peter Lang, 2007), 7–8.

10. Jean-Luc Nancy, *The Inoperative Community,* ed. Peter Conner, trans. Peter Connor, Lisa Garbus, Michael Holland, and Simona Sawhney (Minneapolis: University of Minnesota Press, 1991), 6.

11. Jacques Derrida, *Writing and Difference,* trans. Alan Bass (Chicago: University of Chicago Press, 1978), 71.

12. Jacques Derrida, *Speech and Phenomenon and Other Essays on Husserl's Theory of Signs,* trans. David B. Allison (Evanston, Ill.: Northwestern University Press, 1973), 129–60.

13. Jacques Derrida, *Positions,* trans. Alan Bass (Chicago: University of Chicago Press, 1981), 26, 28.

14. Daniel Callahan, *The Roots of Bioethics: Health, Progress, Technology, Death* (New York: Oxford University Press, 2012), 74.

15. World Health Organization, "Preamble to the Constitution of the World Health Organization," *Official Records of the World Health Organization,* no. 2 (1948): 100. Definition cited at http://www.medical-colleges.net/worldhealth.htm.

16. Karl Jaspers, *Way to Wisdom,* trans. Ralph Manheim (New Haven, Conn: Yale University Press, 1954), 24.

17. Jaspers, *Way to Wisdom,* 125.

18. Kenneth Burke, *Permanence and Change* (New York: Bobbs-Merrill, 1965), 37.

19. The notion of narrative wreckage is adopted from Arthur W. Frank, *The Wounded Storyteller: Body, Illness, and Ethics* (Chicago: University of Chicago Press, 1995).

20. William Earle, *Public Sorrows & Private Pleasures* (Bloomington: Indiana University Press, 1976), 157.

21. My understanding of public moral argument is influenced by Walter R. Fisher, *Human Communication as Narration: Toward a Philosophy of Reason, Value, and Action* (Columbia: University of South Carolina Press, 1987). I say more about Fisher's work later in this introduction.

22. Friedrich Nietzsche, *Twilight of the Idols and The Anti-Christ,* trans. R. J. Hollingdale (New York: Penguin Books, 1990), 33.

23. Kenneth Burke, *Language as Symbolic Action: Essays in Life, Literature, and Method* (Berkeley: University of California Press, 1966), 16.

24. Hans Jonas, *The Phenomenon of Life: Towards a Philosophical Biology* (Chicago: University of Chicago Press, 1966), 175.

25. Cicero, *De oratore* (1.8.32), trans. H. Rackham (Cambridge, Mass.: Harvard University Press, 1942).

26. Ralph Waldo Emerson, *Selections from Ralph Waldo Emerson*, ed. Stephen W. Whicher (Boston: Houghton Mifflin, 1957), 306.

27. Ralph Waldo Emerson, *Nature* (Part IV, "Language"), in *The Essential Writings of Ralph Waldo Emerson,* ed. Brooks Atkinson (New York: Modern Library, 2000), 15; *Essays: First Series* ("Heroism"), in *The Essential Writings,* 228.

28. Northrop Frye, *Fearful Symmetry: A Study of William Blake* (Princeton, N.J.: Princeton University Press, 1969), 236.

29. Annie Dillard, *The Writing Life* (New York: HarperPerennial, 1989), 72.

30. Jaspers, *Way to Wisdom,* 121.

31. Ludwig Wittgenstein, *On Certainty,* trans. Denis Paul and G. E. M. Anscombe (Oxford: Basil Blackwell, 1969–1975), #471.

32. R. Buckminster Fuller, *Intuition* (New York: Anchor Books, 1973), 9–10.

33. Rita Charon, *Narrative Medicine: Honoring the Stories of Illness* (New York: Oxford University Press, 2006), 56, 177.

34. President's Commission for the Study of Bioethical Issues, *Bioethics for Every Generation: Deliberation and Education in Health, Science, and Technology* (Washington, D.C: Presidential Commission for the Study of Bioethical Issues, 2016). Also see King and Hyde (eds.), *Bioethics, Public Moral Argument, and Social Responsibility; Public Deliberation: What It Is and How to Conduct It* (special issue of *The Hastings Center Report*) 42 (March–April 2012); Hyde and Herrick (eds.), *After the Genome;* and Johann A. R. Roduit, *The Case for Perfection: Ethics in the Age of Human Enhancement* (New York: Peter Lang, 2016). Narrative analysis is a well-recognized area of research in health communication and bioethics. The scope of this research is not limited to the physician-patient-family medical encounter. As demonstrated throughout their literature, health communication and bioethics scholars realize that "no narrative is solely personal, organizational or public; stories necessarily bleed across the artificial boundaries of discrete areas of knowledge. Personal stories cannot escape the constraints of institutional interests, nor can they fail to engage the assumptions, expectations, and values encoded in public narratives. Conversely, narratives constructed and circulated in the public domain are built upon personal and institutional narratives drawing from the experiences and understandings of those within their domains." See Phyllis M. Japp, Lynn M. Harter, and Christina S. Beck, "Overview of Narrative and

Health Communication Theorizing," in Lynn M. Harter, Phyllis M. Japp, and Christina S. Beck (eds.), *Narratives, Health, and Healing: Communication Theory, Research, and Practice* (Mahwah, N.J.: Lawrence Erlbaum, 2005), 3. For an excellent review of the health communication literature on narrative analysis up until 2003, see Barbara F. Sharf and Marsha L. Vanderford, "Illness Narratives and the Social Construction of Health," in *Handbook of Health Communication*, eds. Teresa L. Thompson, Alicia M. Dorsey, Katherine I. Miller, and Roxanne Parrot (New York: Taylor & Francis, 2003); and Barbara F. Sharf, Lynn M. Harter, Jill Yamasaki, and Paul Haidet, "Narrative Turns Epic: Contemporary Developments in Health Narrative Scholarship," in *The Routledge Handbook of Health Communication*, eds. Teressa L. Thompson, Roxanne Parrott, and Jon F. Nussbaum (New York: Routledge, 2011), 36–51. Also see Martha Montello (ed), *Narrative Ethics: The Role of Stories in Bioethics*, Special Issue of *The Hastings Center Report* 44 (January–February 2014); and Jim Yamasaki, Patricia Geist-Martin, and Barbara F. Sharf, *Storied Health and Illness: Communicating Personal, Cultural, and Political Complexities* (Long Grove, IL.: Waveland, 2017). What is not found in this literature is the specific study of public moral argument advanced in my story of the interruption that we are. For example, in her essay "The Story Unfolds: Linking Complexities," in *Storied Health and Illness*, 357–79, Patricia Geist-Martin briefly discusses the highly publicized medical aid in dying case of Brittany Maynard, and characterizes the case in general terms as an instance of "personal empowerment constructed through resistance to cultural and political complexities" (376). This is a fair depiction of the case. But Geist-Martin offers no analysis of how the illness story told by Maynard in a number of videos, written statements, and interviews unfolds primarily as an activity of public moral argument. Maynard's story is one of my major case studies. Also see Christina S. Beck, "Becoming the Story: Narratives as Collaborative, Social Enactments of Individual, Relational, and Public Identities," in Harter, Japp, and Beck (eds.), *Narratives, Health, and Healing*, 61–81. Beck offers a case study of a wounded storyteller going public with her illness narrative on cancer. The analysis is not conceived as an event in public moral argument, although Beck does emphasize the rhetorical nature of the narrative.

35. Fisher, *Human Communication as Narration*, 71. For an excellent discussion of the nature, scope, and function of public moral argument and its relevance to bioethics, see David Zarefsky, "Arguing about Values: The Problem of Public Moral Argument," in King and Hyde (eds.), *Bioethics, Public Moral Argument, and Social Responsibility*, 3–13.

36. The King James Version of *The Holy Bible* is used for Scripture quotations throughout my story.

37. The notion of "rotten with perfection" is adopted from Kenneth Burke's influential essay "Definition of Man," in Burke, *Language as Symbolic Action*, 3–24.

38. Ray Kurzweil, *Transcendent Man*, December 8, 2014, http://www.youtube.com/watch?v=R33EzziG5IM.

39. Calvin O. Schrag, *Reflections on the Religious, the Ethical, and the Political*, ed. Michael R. Paradiso-Michau (New York: Lexington Books, 2013), xxxix.

40. Brian Christian, *The Most Human Human: What Artificial Intelligence Teaches Us about Being Alive* (New York: Anchor, 2011), 80.

Chapter 1: The First Interruption

1. Martin Heidegger, *Parmenides,* trans. Andre Schuwer and Richard Rojcewiz (Bloomington: Indiana University Press, 1992), 135–36.

2. Hans-Georg Gadamer, *Truth and Method,* 2nd revised ed., trans. Joel Weinsheimer and Donald G. Marshall (New York: Crossroad, 1989), 299, 363.

3. See, for example, M. Craig Barnes, *When God Interrupts: Finding New Life through Unwanted Change* (Downers Grove, Ill: InterVarsity Press, 1996).

4. Hans Blumenberg, "An Anthropological Approach to the Contemporary Significance of Rhetoric," trans. Robert M. Wallace, in *After Philosophy: End or Transformation,* ed. Kenneth Baynes, James Bohman, and Thomas McCarthy (Cambridge, Mass.: MIT Press, 1987), 441.

5. David J. Wolpe, *In Speech and in Silence* (New York: Henry Holt, 1992), 98.

6. Lawrence Kushner, *God Was in This Place and I, I Did Not Know: Finding Self, Spirituality, and Ultimate Meaning* (Woodstock, Vt.: Jewish Lights, 1991), 31–33.

7. Frederick w. J. Schelling, *Of Human Freedom,* trans. James Gutmann (Chicago: Open Court, 1936), 84.

8. Schelling, *Of Human Freedom,* 84 (emphasis in original).

9. For an excellent discussion and analysis of Luria's life and teachings, see Lawrence Fine, *Physician of the Soul, Healer of the Cosmos: Isaac Luria and His Kabbalistic Fellowship* (Stanford, Calif.: Stanford University Press, 2003). Also see *The Zohar* (Pritzker Edition), trans. and comm. Daniel C. Matt, 3 vols. (Stanford, Calif.: Stanford University Press, 2004–2006).

10. Lawrence Kushner, *The Book of Words: Talking Spiritual Life, Living Spiritual Talk* (Woodstock, Vt.: Jewish Lights, 1993), 28.

11. Marc-Alain Quaknon, *Mysteries of the Kabbalah,* trans. Josephine Bacon (New York: Abbeville Press, 2000), 200.

12. Abraham Joshua Heschel, *God in Search of Man: A Philosophy of Judaism* (New York: Noonday Press, 1955), 136.

13. David A. Cooper, *God Is a Verb: Kabbalah and the Practice of Mystical Judaism* (New York: Riverhead Books, 1997), 43, 58.

14. MJL Staff, "Conversation and Debate: An Overview of the Jewish National Sport: Arguing," *My Jewish Learning,* no date, http://www.myjewishlearning.com/article/conversation-debate/2/.

15. See, for example, Gerald L. Schroeder, *Genesis and the Big Bang: The Discovery of Harmony between Modern Science and the Bible* (New York: Bantam, 1990); John Polkinghorne, *The Faith of a Physicist* (Minneapolis, Minn.: Fortress, 1996); Francis S. Collins, *The Language of God* (New York: Free Press, 2006). I offer a detailed discussion of Collins's book in chapter 7.

16. David Hume, *A Letter from a Gentleman to His Friend in Edinburgh,* ed. Ernest Campbell Mossner and John V. Prince (Edinburgh: Edinburgh University Press, 1967), 25–26.

17. See, for example, William A. Dembski, *Intelligent Design: The Bridge between Science and Theology* (New York: InterVarsity Press, 1999).

18. David Hume, *Essays: Moral, Political, and Literary*, ed. Eugene F. Miller (Indianapolis: Liberty Classics, 1985), 82–83.

19. Hume, *Essays: Moral, Political, and Literary*, 583.

20. Steven Weinberg, *Dreams of a Final Theory: The Scientist's Search for the Ultimate Laws of Nature* (New York: Vintage Books, 1992).

21. Martin Rees, *Before the Beginning: Our Universe and Others* (Reading, Mass.: Perseus Books, 1997), 1.

22. Rees, *Before the Beginning*, 8.

23. Weinberg, *Dreams of a Final Theory*, 242.

24. Richard Feynman, *The Meaning of It All: Thoughts of a Citizen-Scientist* (Reading, Mass.: Perseus Books), 49–50.

25. Steven Weinberg, *Facing Up: Science and Its Cultural Adversaries* (Cambridge, Mass.: Harvard University Press, 2001), 120.

26. References for the present discussion include Paul Davies, *The Cosmic Blueprint: New Discoveries in Nature's Ability to Order the Universe* (Radnor, Pa.: Templeton Foundation Press, 2004); Brian Greene, *The Elegant Universe* (New York: Vintage, 1999); Brian Greene, *The Hidden Reality: Parallel Universes and the Deep Laws of the Cosmos* (New York: Vintage Books, 2011); Alan H. Guth, *The Inflationary Universe: The Quest for a New Theory of Cosmic Origins* (New York: Basic Books, 1998); Stephen W. Hawking, *The Theory of Everything: The Origin and Fate of the Universe* (Beverly Hills, Calif.: 2002); Leon Lederman and Christopher Hill, *Beyond the God Particle* (New York: Prometheus Books, 2013); Lawrence M. Krauss, *A Universe from Nothing: Why Is There Something Rather Than Nothing* (New York: Atria, 2012); Joel R. Primack and Nancy Ellen Abrams, *The View from the Center of the Universe: Discovering Our Extraordinary Place in the Cosmos* (New York: Riverhead Books, 2006); Martin Rees, *Our Cosmic Habitat* (Princeton, N.J.: Princeton University Press, 2001); Rees, *Before the Beginning;* Lee Smolin, *The Life of the Cosmos* (New York: Oxford University Press, 1997) Joseph Silk, *The Big Bang*, 3rd ed. (New York: W. H. Freeman, 2001); Alex Vilenkin, *Many Worlds in One: The Search for Other Universes* (New York: Hill and Wang, 2006); Weinberg, *Dreams of a Final Theory;* Steven Weinberg, *Facing Up: Science and Its Cultural Adversaries* (Cambridge, Mass.: Harvard University Press, 2001); and Steven Weinberg, *The First Three Minutes: A Modern View of the Origin of the Universe*, updated ed. (New York: Basic Books, 1993).

27. Rees, *Our Cosmic Habitat*, 157–81.

28. Paul Davies, *God and the New Physics* (New York: Simon and Schuster, 1983), 70, 209. Also see Paul Davies, *The Fifth Miracle: The Search for the Origins and Meaning of Life* (New York: Simon and Schuster, 2000).

29. Teilhard de Chardin, *The Phenomenon of Man*, 169–70. Religious conservatives would argue, however, that no one can do more than associate with the Divine, since the Divine is perfect and nothing can be added or subtracted if It is to remain perfect. See, for example, Craig R. Smith, *The Quest for Charisma: Christianity and Persuasion* (Westport, Conn.: Praeger, 2000).

30. Lewis Thomas, "The Wonderful Mistake," in *Being Human: Core Readings in the Humanities*, ed. Leon Kass (New York: W. W. Norton, 2004), 31–32.

31. Thomas, "The Wonderful Mistake," 32.

32. Thomas, "The Wonderful Mistake," 32.

33. Thomas, "The Wonderful Mistake," 32–33.

34. Lee Smolin, *Time Reborn: From the Crisis in Physics to the Future of the Universe* (New York: Mariner Books, 2014), xiv.

Chapter 2: Existence and the Self

1. Michael Mallary, *Our Improbable Universe: A Physicist Considers How We Got Here* (New York: Thunder's Mouth Press, 2004), 177, 180.

2. Søren Kierkegaard, *Provocations*, ed. Charles Moore (New York: Orbis Books, 2005), 263.

3. Søren Kierkegaard, *Either/Or*, vol. 2, trans. David F. Swenson and Lillian Marvin Swenson (Princeton, N.J.: Princeton University Press, 1971), 364.

4. Søren Kierkegaard, *Concluding Unscientific Postscript*, trans. D. F. Swenson and W. Lowrie (Princeton, N.J.: Princeton University Press, 1971), 279.

5. Kierkegaard, *Concluding Unscientific Postscript*, 327.

6. Kierkegaard, *Concluding Unscientific Postscript*, 393.

7. Kierkegaard, *Provocations*, 263.

8. Vladimir Nabokov, "The Art of Literature and Common Sense," in *Lectures on Literature*, ed. Fredson Bowers (New York: Mariner Books, 2002), 372.

9. Søren Kierkegaard, *The Point of View for My Work as an Author: A Report to History and Related Writings*, trans. Walter Lowrie, ed. Benjamin Nelson (New York: Harper Torchbooks, 1962), 112.

10. Kierkegaard, *Provocations*, 244.

11. Paul Brockelman, *Time and Self: Phenomenological Explorations* (New York: Crossroad, 1985), 12.

12. Kierkegaard, *Concluding Unscientific Postscript*, 147.

13. Søren Kierkegaard, *Christian Discourses*, trans. Walter Lowrie (New York: Oxford University Press, 1939), 80.

14. Kierkegaard, *Either/Or*, 146.

15. Søren Kierkegaard, *Either/Or*, vol. 1, trans. David F. Swenson and Lillian Marvin Swenson (Princeton, NJ.: Princeton University Press, 1977), 188. Further references to the story of Elvira are cited in the text.

16. Søren Kierkegaard, *Fear and Trembling* and *The Sickness unto Death*, trans. Walter Lowrie (Princeton, N.J..: Princeton University Press, 1941), 30.

17. Søren Kierkegaard, *The Concept of Dread*, trans. Walter Lowrie (Princeton, N.J.: Princeton University Press, 1957), 139.

18. Quoted in Carl Elliott, *Better Than Well: American Medicine Meets the American Dream* (New York: W. W. Norton, 2003), 75.

19. Ann Pietrangelo, "Recognizing Anxiety: Symptoms, Signs, and Risk Fact," *Health Line*, September 24, 2014, http://www.healthline.com/health/anxiety/effects-on-body.

20. Jacques Derrida, "Deconstruction and the Other," in *Dialogues with Contemporary Continental Thinkers: The Phenomenological Heritage*, ed. R. Kearney (Manchester: Manchester University Press, 1984), 116, 120.

21. Jacques Derrida, "Afterword: Toward an Ethic of Discussion," trans. S. Weber, in *Jacques Derrida, Limited Inc.*, trans. S. Weber and J. Mehlman (Evanston, Ill.: Northwestern University Press, 1988), 147.

22. Kierkegaard, *Concluding Unscientific Postscript,* 169.

23. Kierkegaard, *Concluding Unscientific Postscript,* 244.

24. Kierkegaard, *Concluding Unscientific Postscript,* 265.

25. Kierkegaard, *Concluding Unscientific Postscript,* 69.

26. Kierkegaard, *Fear and Trembling and The Sickness unto Death,* 146.

27. Woody Allen, *Getting Even* (New York: Vintage, 1978), 21.

28. Saint Augustine, *Confessions* (III.iv.7–8), trans. Henry Chadwick (New York: Oxford University Press, 1992).

29. Augustine, *On Christian Doctrine* (4.III.5), trans. D. W. Robertson, Jr. (Upper Saddle River, N.J.: Prentice Hall).

30. Heiko Schulz, "Eloquence, Faith and Probability," in *Kierkegaard and the Greek World, Tome II: Aristotle and Other Greek Authors,* ed. Jon Stewart and Katalin Nun (West Court East, London, England: Ashgate, 2010), 96.

31. Kierkegaard, *Provocations,* 244.

32. Cicero, *De officiis* (1:7:22; 1.6:19), trans. Walter Miller (Cambridge, Mass.: Harvard University Press, 1913).

33. Søren Kierkegaard, *The Concept of Anxiety: A Simple Psychologically Orienting Deliberation on the Dogmatic Issue of Hereditary Sin,* trans. and ed. Reidar Thomte, in collaboration with Albert B. Anderson (Princeton, N.J.: Princeton University Press, 1980), 188.

34. Søren Kierkegaard, *The Book of Adler,* trans. Howard V. Hong and Edna H. Hong (Princeton, N.J.: Princeton University Press, 1998), 92.

35. Søren Kierkegaard, "Freedom of Conscience, Freedom of Belief," *The Journals of Kierkegaard,* trans. Alexander Dru (New York: Harper and Brothers, 1959), 185.

36. Martin Heidegger, "Letter on Humanism," trans. Frank A. Capuzzi, in collaboration with J. Glenn Gray, in *Basic Writings,* ed. David Farrell Krell (New York: Harper and Row, 1977), 230.

37. Heidegger, *Being and Time,* 32.

38. Martin Heidegger, *An Introduction to Metaphysics,* trans. Ralph Mannheim (New Haven, Conn.: Yale University Press, 1959), 205.

39. Heidegger, *Being and Time,* 95–107

40. Heidegger, *Being and Time,* 164–65.

41. Heidegger, *Being and Time,* 177–78.

42. Heidegger, *Being and Time,* 67, 163–68, 369.

43. The distinction I am making here between the call of conscience and the interruption that we are is not specified by Heidegger.

44. Heidegger, "Letter on Humanism," 237.

45. See, for example, Martin Heidegger, *What Is Called Thinking?,* trans. J. Glenn Gray (New York: Harper and Row, 1968), 37–41, 138–47.

46. Heidegger, *Being and Time,* 321–22.

47. Heidegger, *Being and Time,* 316.

48. Heidegger, *Being and Time,* 233, 279–311.

49. Heidegger, *Being and Time,* 358. Jerry Shaw, "Positive Effects of Anxiety," *Livestrong.com,* December 5, 2015, http://www.livestrong.com/article/228293-positive-effects-of-anxiety/; Nancy C. Andreasen, "The Relationship between Creativity and Mood Disorders," *Clinical Neuroscience* 2 (2008): 251–55.

50. Heidegger, *Being and Time,* 311, 422, 437.

51. Heidegger, *Being and Time,* 344–45. Heidegger acknowledges that Being-with-others is an inevitable condition of one's life. Even being "alone" presupposes a Being-with-others, for an individual can be alone only because the other is not present. "So far as [human being] is at all," writes Heidegger, "it has Being-with-one-another as its kind of Being" (163). What an individual is now in her life carries with it a history that has "always already" been influenced by the other. Human existence is marked with an indelible communal character.

52. Martin Heidegger, *Existence and Being,* trans. Douglas Scott, R. F. C. Hull, and Alan Crick (South Bend, Ind.: Henry Regnery, 1949), 275.

53. Heidegger, *Being and Time,* 355, 436.

54. Heidegger, *Being and Time,* 158–59.

55. Heidegger, *Being and Time,* 206. For an exceptional assessment of the virtue of listening, see Lisbeth Lipari, *Listening, Thinking, Being: Toward an Ethics of Attunement* (University Park; The Pennsylvania State University Press, 2014).

56. Robert N. Bellah, R. Madsen, W. M. Sullivan, A. Swidler, and S. M. Tipton, *Habits of the Heart: Individualism and Commitment in American Life* (New York: Harper and Row, 1985), 162, 251.

57. Henry W. Johnstone Jr., *Philosophy and Argument* (University Park: Pennsylvania State University Press, 1959), 19.

58. Henry W. Johnstone Jr., *Validity and Rhetoric in Philosophical Argument: An Outlook in Transition* (University Park, Pa.: Dialogue Press, 1978), 129.

59. Martin Heidegger, *Grundbegriffe der Aristotelischen Phiosophie: Marburger Vorlesung Summersemester 1924, Gesamtausgabe,* vol. 18, ed. Mark Michalski (Frankfurt: Klostermann, 2002).

60. Nancy S. Struever, "Alltäglichkeit, Timefulness, in the Heideggerian Program," in *Heidegger and Rhetoric,* ed. Daniel M. Gross and Ansgar Kemmann (New York: State University of New York Press, 2005), 127.

61. Martin Heidegger, "Rectorial Address: The Self-Assertion of the German University," in *Martin Heidegger and National Socialism,* ed. Gunther Neske and Emil Kettering (New York: Paragon House, 1990), 5–13. Further references to this address will be cited in the text.

62. Heidegger, *An Introduction to Metaphysics,* 199.

63. Heidegger, *An Introduction to Metaphysics,* 61–62. For an excellent discussion of Heraclitus, see Charles H. Kahn, *The Art and Thought of Heraclitus: An Edition of the Fragments with Translation and Commentary* (New York: Cambridge University Press, 1979).

64. Hans Sluga, *Heidegger's Crisis: Philosophy and Politics in Nazi Germany* (Cambridge, Mass.: Harvard University Press, 1993), 197–98.

65. See, for example, Jean-Francois Lyotard, *Heidegger and "the Jews,"* trans. Andreas

Michel and Mark S. Roberts (Minneapolis: University of Minnesota Press, 1990); Richard Wolin, *The Politics of Being, The Political Thought of Martin Heidegger* (New York: Columbia University Press, 1990); Berel Lang, *Heidegger's Silence* (Ithaca, N.Y.: Cornell University Press, 1996); Alan Milchman and Alan Rosenberg (eds.), *Martin Heidegger and the Holocaust* (Atlantic Highlands, N.J.: Humanities Press, 1996).

66. Cited in Wolin, *The Politics of Being,* 168.

67. Martin Heidegger, "The Rectorate 1933/34: Facts and Thoughts," trans. Lisa Harries, in *Martin Heidegger and National Socialism,* ed. Gunther Neske and Emil Kettering (New York: Paragon House, 1990), 15–32.

68. Martin Heidegger, *Reading Heidegger's Black Notebooks 1931–1941,* ed. Ingo Farin and Jeff Malpas (Cambridge, Mass.: MIT Press, 2016).

69. Adolph Hitler, *Mein Kampf,* trans. Ralph Manheim (New York: Houghton Mifflin, 1998), 296.

70. Emmanuel Levinas, *Ethics and Infinity,* trans. Richard A. Cohen (Pittsburgh, Pa.: Duquesne University Press, 1985), 42.

71. For the book that offers what I consider to be the most fair-minded assessment of Heidegger's philosophical accomplishments and mind-numbing political failures, see Rudiger Safranski, *Martin Heidegger: Between Good and Evil,* trans. Ewald Osers (Cambridge, Mass.: Harvard University Press, 1998). Also see, for example, Michael E. Zimmerman, *Heidegger's Confrontation with Modernity: Technology, Politics, Art* (Bloomington: Indiana University Press, 1990); Hubert L. Dreyfus and Harrison Hall, *Heidegger: A Critical Reader* (Oxford: Basil Blackwell, 1992); George Steiner, *Martin Heidegger* (Chicago: University of Chicago Press, 1978). These works contain critiques of Heidegger that speak of his association with National Socialism in ways that undoubtedly will be repeated and advanced in publications reacting to Heidegger's *Black Book Diaries.* The "Heidegger Debate" has become a permanent event in the history of contemporary philosophy.

Chapter 3: Existence and the Other

1. Abraham Joshua Heschel, *Man Is Not Alone: A Philosophy of Religion* (New York: Noonday Press, 1951), 296.

2. Emmanuel Levinas, *Time and the Other,* trans. Richard Cohen (Pittsburgh, Pa.: Duquesne University Press, 1987), 58.

3. Levinas, *Time and the Other,* 42.

4. Emmanuel Levinas, *Existence and Existents,* trans. Alphonso Lingis (The Hague: Martinus Nijhoff, 1978), 23.

5. Levinas, *Time and the Other,* 54.

6. Levinas, *Time and the Other,* 55.

7. Levinas, *Time and the Other,* 69.

8. Levinas, *Time and the Other,* 55.

9. Emmanuel Levinas, *Totality and Infinity,* trans. Alphonso Lingis (Pittsburg, PA.: Duquesne University Press, 1969), 144–45.

10. Levinas, *Ethics and Infinity,* trans. Richard Cohen (Pittsburgh, Pa.: Duquesne University Press, 1985), 97.

11. Emmanuel Levinas, *Collected Philosophical Papers,* trans. Alphonso Lingis (The Hague: Martinus Nijhoff, 1987), 20.

12. Abraham Joshua Heschel, *I Asked for Wonder: A Spiritual Anthology,* ed. Samuel H. Dresner (New York: Crossroad, 1997), 48

13. Levinas, *Ethics and Infinity,* 87.

14. Emmanuel Levinas, "Ethics of the Infinite" (Interview with Richard Kearney), in *Dialogues with Contemporary Continental Thinkers: The Phenomenological Heritage,* ed. Richard Kearney (Manchester, UK: Manchester University Press, 1984), 62–63.

15. Emmanuel Levinas, *Outside the Subject,* trans. Michael B. Smith (Stanford, Calif.: Stanford University Press, 1994), 135–43.

16. Diane Davis, *Inessential Solidarity: Rhetoric and Foreigner Relations* (Pittsburgh, Pa.: University of Pittsburgh, 2010), 56–57, 111. For a discussion of how the rhetoric of the face *is* a primordial form of eloquence, see Michael J. Hyde, *The Call of Conscience: Heidegger and Levinas, Rhetoric and the Euthanasia Debate* (Columbia: University of South Carolina Press, 2001), 79–115.

17. Emmanuel Levinas, *Difficult Freedom: Essays on Judaism,* trans. Sean Hand (Baltimore, Md.: Johns Hopkins University Press, 1990), 9–10.

18. Levinas, *Ethics and Infinity,* 105–6.

19. Emmanuel Levinas, *Otherwise Than Being or Beyond Essence,* trans. Alphonso Lingis (Boston: Klumer, 1991), 38. For an excellent work on Levinas that makes much of this point see Amit Pinchevski, *By Way of Interruption: Levinas and the Ethics of Communication* (Pittsburgh, Pa.: Duquesne University Press, 2005).

20. Emmanuel Levinas, "Ethics as First Philosophy," in Emmanuel Levinas, *The Levinas Reader,* ed. Sean Hand (Oxford: Blackwell, 1989), 83.

21. Levinas, *Totality and Infinity,* 197–201, 246, 262, 303.

22. Levinas, *Collected Philosophical Papers,* 148.

23. Levinas, *Time and the Other, 56.*

24. Levinas, *Time and the Other,* 137.

25. Emmanuel Levinas, *Alterity & Transcendence,* trans. Michael B. Smith (New York: Columbia University Press, 1999), 97.

26. Levinas, *Otherwise Than Being,* 158.

27. Emmanuel Levinas, *Entre Nous: Thinking-of-the-Other,* trans. Michael B. Smith and Barbara Harshav (New York: Columbia University Press, 1998), 105.

28. Emmanuel Levinas and Richard Kearney, "Dialogue with Emmanuel Levinas," in *Face to Face with Levinas,* ed. Richard A. Cohen (New York: State University of New York Press, 1986), 32–33.

29. Wilbur S. Howell (ed.), *Fenelon's Dialogues on Eloquence* (Princeton, N.J.: Princeton University Press, 1951), 23.

30. Kenneth Burke, *Counter-Statement* (Berkeley: University of California Press, 1968), 167. The classic discussion of eloquence in the rhetorical tradition is Cicero's *Orator,* trans. H. M. Hubbell (Cambridge, Mass.: Harvard University Press, 1962).

31. Levinas, *Totality and Infinity,* 72; Emmanuel Levinas, *Outside the Subject,* trans. Michael B. Smith (Stanford, Calif.: Stanford University Press, 1994), 138–39.

32. Levinas, *Outside the Subject,* 138–39.

33. Hans-Georg Gadamer, *Truth and Method,* 2nd revised ed., trans. Joel Weinsheimer and Donald G. Marshall (New York: Crossroad, 1989), 383.

34. Calvin O. Schrag, *Communicative Praxis and the Space of Subjectivity* (Bloomington: Indiana University Press, 1986), 198–99.

35. The radio discussion is contained in Levinas, *The Levinas Reader,* 289–97. Further references to this discussion are contained in the text.

36. Slavoj Zizek, *Organs without Bodies: Deleuze and Consequences* (New York: Routledge, 2003), 106.

37. Georges Gusdorf, *Speaking (La Parole),* trans. Paul T. Brockelman (Evanston, Ill.: Northwestern University Press, 1965), 47.

38. Etty Hillesum, *An Interrupted Life: The Diaries, 1941–1943 and Letters from Westerbork,* trans. Arnold J. Pomerans (New York: Henry Holt, 1996). Further references to this work will be cited in the text.

39. Heschel, *Man Is Not Alone,* 193–95.

40. Levinas, *Time and the Other,* 114.

41. Heschel, *I Asked for Wonder,* 72.

42. See, for example, Levinas, *Totality and Infinity,* 257–59; Levinas, *Collected Philosophical Papers,* 121–24; Levinas, *Otherwise Than Being,* 146–47.

43. Søren Kierkegaard, *Concluding Unscientific Postscript,* trans. D. F. Swenson and W. Lowrie (Princeton, N.J.: Princeton University Press, 1971), 279.

44. Charles Siebert, "The Rehumanization of the Heart: What Doctors Have Forgotten, Poets Have Always Known," *Harper's* (February 1990), 53–60; Charles Siebert, *A Man after His Own Heart* (New York: Crown, 2004). Further references to these works are contained in the text. The essay is noted with an "R." The book is noted with an "M."

45. Renee C. Fox and Judith P. Swazey, *Spare Parts: Organ Replacement in American Society* (New Brunswick, N.J.: Transaction, 2013), 161–62.

46. Eric J. Cassell, *The Nature of Suffering and the Goals of Medicine* (New York: Oxford University Press, 1991), 167. For an excellent study that makes much of this point, see Lisa Keränen, *Scientific Characters: Rhetoric, Politics, and Trust in Breast Cancer Research* (Tuscaloosa: University of Alabama Press, 2010).

Chapter 4: The Right Word

1. W. H. S. Jones, *Hippocrates,* vol. 2: *Law* (London: William Heinemann; New York: G. P. Putnam's Sons, 1923), iv.

2. Anatole Broyard, *Intoxicated by My Illness and Other Writings on Life and Death* (New York: Fawcett Columbine, 1992), 19–20, 50.

3. Arthur W. Frank, *The Wounded Storyteller: Body, Illness, and Ethics* (Chicago: University of Chicago Press, 1995), 17.

4. Frank, *The Wounded Storyteller,* 17–18.

5. Frank, *The Wounded Storyteller,* 56. For a must read extension of Frank's work, see Kathlyn Conway's *Beyond Words: Illness and the Limits of Expression* (Albuquerque: University of New Mexicao Press, 2007). Conway, a practicing psychotherapist and cancer survivor, offers an exceptionally lucid and original analysis of narratives whose authors focus specially on the pain and suffering associated with their various

illnesses. Conway writes: "I and many who are ill and disabled have longed for a story that takes us into the darker and less familiar corners of the territory of illness, what Reynolds Price calls 'the far side of catastrophe, the dim other side of that high wall that effectively shuts disaster off from the unfazed world' [Reynolds Price, *A Whole New Life* (New York: Scribners Classics, 1994), 180]. It is a world unto itself, and we who find ourselves there discover that the usual resources for coping are sorely tried. We long to hear from someone who speaks from within personal experience and describes what it is really like to have cancer, to lose a leg, to become blind, or to feel the mind spinning out of control. We long to hear from someone who admits that even enormous love from others does not erase the essential loneliness of illness. We want to hear not clichés but an acknowledgment that illness is not simply an opportunity for personal growth but a soul-wrenching encounter with loss, limitation, and the reality of death. We want to hear from someone who does not go gently into that dark night" (2). Conway offers a brief discussion (113–17) of how interruption can be used to construct a narrative that exposes what she wants to hear about illness. Her two examples are Virginia Woolf's essay "On Being Ill" (1930) and Donald Hall's *Life Work* (1993). Neither of these literary works, however, have as their primary goal the advancement of public moral argument.

6. Gusdorf, *Speaking (La Parole),* 125.

7. Danielle Ofir, *What Doctors Feel: How Emotions Affect the Practice of Medicine* (New York: Beacon Press, 2014); Tamara Sims and Jeanne L. Tsai, "Patients Respond More Positively to Physicians Who Focus on Their Ideal Affect," *Emotion* 15 (June 2015): 303–18; John Heritage and Anna Lindström, "Knowledge, Empathy and Emotion in a Medical Encounter," in *Emotion and Affect in Interaction,* ed. Anssi Peräkylä and Marja-Leena Sorjonen (Oxford: Oxford University Press, 2012), 256–73.

8. Ralph Crawshaw, "Technical Zeal or Therapeutic Purpose—How to Decide?," *Journal of the American Medical Association* 250 (1983): 1859. Also see Robert Wachter, *The Digital Doctor: Hope, Hype, and Harm at the Dawn of Medicine's Computer Age* (New York: McGraw-Hill, 2015).

9. Kenneth Burke, *Permanence and Change: An Anatomy of Purpose* (New York: Bobbs-Merrill, 1965), 79, 44–47.

10. Kenneth Burke, *Language as Symbolic Action: Essays in Life, Literature, and Method* (Berkeley: University of California Press, 1966), 19.

11. *Seinfeld,* "The Opposite," episode no. 86, first broadcast May 19, 1994, by NBC. Directed by Thom Cherones and written by Andy Cowan, Larry David, and Jerry Seinfeld.

12. The heart symbol, the popular icon for the heart associated with Valentine's Day, can be traced to before the last Ice Age (10,000–8,000 B.C.E.). Cro-Magnon hunters in Europe used the symbol in pictograms etched on cave walls. It is not possible, however, to determine the intended meaning of the pictograms since writing had yet to be invented.

13. Arthur Conan Doyle, "A Scandal in Bohemia," in *The Complete Original Illustrated Sherlock Holmes* (Secaucus, N.J.: Castle Books, 1976), 11.

14. Denise M. Duelzinski and Carrol Ahatez, "Repairing 'Difficult' Patient-Clinician Relationships," *AMA Journal of Ethics* 19 (2017): 364–68.

15. Renee C. Fox and Judith P. Swazey, *Spare Parts: Organ Replacement in American Society* (New Brunswick, N.J.: Transaction, 2013), 160. For one of the first discussions of the history and promise of the artificial heart program, see Barton J. Bernstein, "The Pursuit of the Artificial Heart," *Medical Heritage* 2 (March/April 1986): 80–100.

16. Emmanuel Levinas, *Time and the Other,* trans. Richard Cohen (Pittsburgh, Pa.: Duquesne University Press, 1987), 114.

17. http://en.wikipedia.org/wiki/William_J._Schroeder.

18. Rivers Singleton Jr., Letters to the Editor. "Artificial Heart: William Schroeder Was Victim." August 25, 1986, http://articles.philly.com/1986-08-25/news/26064379_1_artificial-heart-artificial-heart-program-william-schroeder.

19. Fox and Swazey, *Spare Parts,* 192–93.

20. Federal Food and Drug Administration, "FDA Approves First Totally Implanted Permanent Artificial Heart for Humanitarian Uses," September 5, 2006, http://www.fda.gov/NewsEvents/Newsroom/PressAnnouncements/2006/ucm108724.htm.

21. Gino Geyosa, "Present and Future Perspectives on Total Artificial Hearts," *Annals of Cardiothoracic Surgery* 6 (2014): 595–162; Joaquin Palomino, "The Heart is Just a Pump," *The Verge,* 2015, https:www.theverge.com/2015/11/4/9665904.artificial/heart-transplant, June 8, 2017; Syncardio Systems, "Press Releases," 2017, www.syncardia.com/2017-press-releases/intex.html, April 10, 2017.

Chapter 5: The Self as Other, the Other as Self

1. Mary Johnson, *Clint Eastwood, Christopher Reeve, and the Case against Disability Rights* (New York: Advocado Press, 2003); Dana S. Dunn, *The Social Psychology of Disability* (New York: Oxford University Press, 2015).

2. Arthur W. Frank, *The Wounded Storyteller: Body, Illness, and Ethics* (Chicago: University of Chicago Press, 1995), 25.

3. Cited in Wesley J. Smith, *Culture of Death: The Assault on Medical Ethics in America* (San Francisco: Encounter Books, 2000), 28.

4. Friedrich Nietzsche, *Twilight of the Idols/The Anti-Christ,* trans. R. J. Hollingdale (New York: Penguin, 1990), 99–100.

5. Hans Blumenberg, "An Anthropological Approach to the Contemporary Significance of Rhetoric," trans. Robert M. Wallace, in *After Philosophy: End or Transformation,* ed. Kenneth Baynes, James Bohman, and Thomas McCarthy (Cambridge, Mass.: MIT Press, 1987), 442.

6. Peter Singer, *Practical Ethics,* 3rd ed. (New York: Cambridge University Press, 2011), 13–14. This book is my major source of data for appreciating Singer's arguments on relevant topics. Helpful preparation for understanding these arguments is offered in Peter Singer, *Rethinking Life and Death: The Collapse of Our Traditional Ethics* (New York: St. Martin's Press, 1994). Here Singer develops a "new" ethics intended to replace the "old" ethics wherein the doctrine of the "sanctity of life" is emphasized. His five "commandments" include: "Recognize that the worth of human life varies"; "Take responsibility for the consequence of your decisions"; "Respect a person's desire to live or die"; "Bring children into the world only if they are wanted"; "Do not discriminate on the basis of species." I offer a more detailed discussion of Singer's philosophy as I continue to review Johnson's story.

7. Henry W. Johnstone Jr., "Some Reflections on Argumentation," in *Philosophy, Rhetoric, and Argumentation,* ed. Maurice Natanson and Henry W. Johnstone Jr. (University Park: Pennsylvania State University Press, 1965), 4–5.

8. Johnstone, "Some Reflections on Argumentation," 7.

9. http://www.nytimes.com/2003/02/16/magazine/unspeakable-conversations.html. Further references to this essay will be cited in the text.

10. See, for example, http://notdeadyet.org/about.

11. Georges Gusdorf, *Speaking* (*La Parole*), trans. Paul T. Brockelman (Evanston, Ill.: Northwestern University Press, 1965), 74–75.

12. http://en.wikipedia.org/wiki/Harriet_McBryde_Johnson.

13. Eric J. Cassell, *The Nature of Suffering and the Goals of Medicine* (New York: Oxford University Press, 1991), 167.

14. MetroWest Center of Independent Living, http://www.mwcil.org/ilhist/leaders/johnson.

15. Singer, *Practical Ethics,* 152.

16. Singer, *Practical Ethics,* 77

17. Elaine Scarry, *On Beauty and Being Just* (Princeton, N.J.: Princeton University Press, 1999), 52–53.

18. Scarry, *On Beauty and Being Just,* 28, 69, 109.

19. Johann Hari, "Peter Singer: Some People Are More Equal Than Others," *The Independent,* July 1, 2004, http://www.independent.co.uk/news/people/profiles/peter-singer-some-people-are-more-equal-than-others-6166342.html.

20. Hari, "Peter Singer: Some People Are More Equal Than Others."

21. Quoted in Stephen Drake, "Peter Singer's 'Tribute' to Harriet Johnson—and Paul Longmore's Response," January 13, 2009, http://notdeadyet.org/2009/01/peter-singers-tribute-to-harriet.html.

22. Peter Singer, "Happy Nevertheless," December 24, 2008, http://www.nytimes.com/2008/12/28/magazine/28mcbryde-t.html.

Chapter 6: A Good Showing of a Bad Situation

1. Heidi EarthBound TomBoy, "The World Needs More Heroes," October 23, 2014, http://earthboundtomboy.blogspot.com/2014/10/the-world-needs-more-heroes.html.

2. Consider, for example, Oregon's requirements: The Death with Dignity Act (ORS §§ 127.800 to 127.897) allows terminally ill Oregon residents to obtain and use prescriptions from their physicians for self-administered lethal medications. Under the act, ending one's life in accordance with the law does not constitute suicide. However, the law is referred to as "physician-assisted suicide" because it allows people to end their lives through the voluntary self-administration of lethal medications prescribed by a physician for that purpose. The Death with Dignity Act legalizes physician-assisted suicide but specifically prohibits euthanasia, in which a physician or other person directly administers a medication to end another's life. The Death with Dignity Act requires that to request a prescription for lethal medications, a patient must voluntarily express his wish to die and be:

1. an adult (age 18 or older),
2. an Oregon resident,
3. capable (able to make and communicate health-care decisions), and
4. diagnosed with a terminal illness (incurable and irreversible) that will lead to death within six months.

Patients meeting these requirements are eligible to request a prescription for lethal medication from a licensed Oregon physician. To receive a prescription for lethal medication, the following steps must be fulfilled:

1. the patient must make two oral requests to his physician, separated by at least 15 days;
2. the patient must provide a written, witnessed request to his physician (two witnesses);
3. the prescribing physician and a consulting physician must confirm the diagnosis and prognosis;
4. the prescribing physician and a consulting physician must determine whether the patient is capable;
5. if either physician believes the patient's judgment is impaired by a psychiatric or psychological disorder, he must refer the patient for a psychological examination;
6. the prescribing physician must inform the patient of feasible alternatives to assisted suicide, including comfort care, hospice care, and pain control; and
7. the prescribing physician must request but may not require the patient to notify his next of kin of the prescription request.

To comply with the law, physicians must report to Oregon Health Services (OHS) all prescriptions for lethal medications. Reporting is not required if patients begin the request process but never receive a prescription. Physicians must inform pharmacists of the prescribed medication's ultimate use. Physicians and patients who adhere to the act's requirements are protected from criminal prosecution, and the choice of legal physician-assisted suicide cannot affect the status of a patient's health or life insurance policies. Physicians and health-care systems are under no obligation to participate in the Death with Dignity Act. https://public.health.oregon.gov/.../DeathwithDignityAct/.../requirements.pdf.

3. Peter Singer, *Practical Ethics,* 3rd ed. (New York: Cambridge University Press, 2011), 170.

4. *Ability Rights Magazine,* "Harriet McBryde Johnson: Civil Rights Activist," http://www.abilitymagazine.com/harriet_mcbryde.html, February 16, 2003.

5. Ronald M. Green, "Good Rules Have Good Reasons: A Response to Leon Kass," in *A Time to Be Born and a Time to Die,* ed. Barry S. Kogan (New York: Aldine de Gruyter, 1991), 152.

6. Martin Foss, *Death, Sacrifice, and Tragedy* (Lincoln: University of Nebraska Press, 1966), 43.

7. Leon R. Kass, "Death with Dignity and the Sanctity of Life," in Kogan, ed., *A Time to Be Born and a Time to Die,* 137.

8. Kass, "Death with Dignity and the Sanctity of Life," 137.

9. For supportive assessments of this position offered by a physician, see Timothy E. Quill, *Death and Dignity: Making Choices and Taking Charge* (New York: W. W. Norton, 1993); Timothy E. Quill, *A Midwife through the Dying Process: Stories of Healing and Hard Choices at the End of Life* (Baltimore, Md.: Johns Hopkins University Press, 1996).

10. Emmanual Levinas, *Time and the Other,* trans. Richard Cohen (Pittsburgh, Pa.: Duquesne University Press, 1987), 109.

11. During a phone interview on April 26, 2016, with Maynard's husband, Dan Diaz, I was told that Maynard favored the term "medical aid in dying" to describe her cause. I thus use the term throughout my discussion out of respect for Maynard and Diaz.

12. See The Brittany Fund, October 6, 2014, https://www.youtube.com/watch?v=yPfe3rCcUeQ, October 6, 2014.

13. Quoted in Jessica Durando, "Brittany Maynard, Right-to-Die Advocate, Ends Her Life," *USA Today Network,* November 3, 2014, http://www.usatoday.com/story/news/nation-now/2014/11/02/brittany-maynard-/18390069/.

14. Natasha Lennard, "29-Year-Old Brittany Maynard's Suicide Was Heroic," November 3, 2014, https://news.vice.com/article/29-year-old-brittany-maynards-suicide-was-heroic.

15. Rhetorical scholars have followed developments in the euthanasia debate for some time. See, for example, Michael J. Hyde, *The Call of Conscience* (Columbia: University of South Carolina Press, 2001), esp. 124–263; Robert Wade Kenny, "A Cycle of Terms Implicit in the Idea of Medicine: Karen Ann Quinlan as a Rhetorical Icon and the Transvaluation of the Ethics of Euthanasia," *Health Communication* 17 (2005): 17–39; Judy Segal, *Health and the Rhetoric of Medicine* (Carbondale: Southern Illinois University Press, 2005); Ellen Bardon, "Situating End-of-Life Decision-Making in a Hybrid Ethical Frame," *Communication and Medicine* 4 (2007): 131–40; Megan Foley, "Voicing Terri Schiavo: Pzrosopopec Citizenship in the Democratic Aporia between Sovereignty and Biopower," *Communication and Critical Cultural Studies* 7 (2010): 381–400; Michael J. Hyde, *Perfection: Coming to Terms with Being Human* (Waco, Tex.: Baylor University Press, 2010), esp. 181–210; Stuart Chambers, "Why Suffering Children Should Have the Right to Assisted Dying," *Ottawa Citizen* (March 2, 2016), http://ottawacitizen.com/opinion/columnists/chambers-why-suffering-children-should-have-the-right-to-assisted-dying.

16. R. Buckminster Fuller, *Intuition* (New York: Anchor Books, 1973), 10.

17. *The Meredith Vieira Show,* "Did Brittany Maynard Have Second Thoughts?," January 14, 2015, https://www.youtube.com/watch?v=AqGVigMakf4.

18. Henry W. Johnstone Jr., *Validity and Rhetoric in Philosophical Argument: An Outlook in Transition* (University Park, Pa.: Dialogue Press, 1978), 129.

19. Burke is known for associating his notion of perspective by incongruity with what he terms the "comic frame." Burke's use of this notion, however, is also applied to rhetorical matters that are not geared to learning by laughter. See Kenneth Burke, *Permanence and Change: An Anatomy of Purpose* (New York: Bobbs-Merrill, 1965).

20. Brittany Maynard, "A New Video for My Friends," October 29, 2014, https://www.youtube.com/watch?v=1lHXHoZb2QI.

21. Anatole Broyard, *Intoxicated by My Illness and Other Writings on Life and Death* (New York: Fawcett Columbine, 1992), 20.

22. Kenneth Burke, *Counter-Statement* (Berkeley: University of California Press, 1968), 167.

23. The plain style differs dramatically from the "grand style" of eloquence and less so from the "middle style" of eloquence. Put simply, the grand style relies heavily on figurative language and is thus commonly associated with the opulent, ornate, and beautiful composition of words. The grand orator is fiery and impetuous; his eloquence, as Cicero puts it, "rushes along with the roar of a mighty stream." The middle style "avoids the fiery force" of the grand style. It makes a moderate use of figurative language, and its diction and rhythm can be poetic. Its sentences can be elaborate and ornate. Its chief virtue is pleasure. Cicero, *Orator,* trans. H. M. Hubbell (Cambridge, Mass.: Harvard University Press, 1988), v. 19–viii 27; xxviii. 97–99.

24. Georges Gusdorf, *Speaking (La Parole),* trans. Paul T. Brockelman (Evanston, Ill.: Northwestern University Press, 1965), 75–76.

25. Marcus Tullius Cicero, *Cicero's Three Books of Offices,* trans. Cyrus R. Edmonds (Cambridge: H. G. Bohn, 1856), 197–98.

26. Kenneth Burke, *Counter-Statement* (Berkeley: University of California Press, 1968), 169–70.

27. Jürgen Habermas, *Moral Consciousness and Communicative Action,* trans. Christian Lenhardt and Shierry Weber Nicholsen (Cambridge, Mass.: MIT Press, 1990).

28. Alison (Sunny) Maynard, a woman claiming to be Brittany's aunt, argues that the Brittany in the original Compassion & Choices video, TV interviews, and magazine photos is a fake planted by the "CIA/media hoax network" to induce the public "to expand availability of assisted suicide." Alison Maynard, "Brittany Maynard, My Undead Niece," *The Real Colorado,* http://therealcolorado.blogspot.com/2015/02/brittany-maynard-my-undead-niece.html.

29. Brittany Maynard," My Right to Death with Dignity at 29," *CNN,* November 2, 2014, http://www.cnn.com/2014/10/07/opinion/maynard-assisted-suicide-cancer-dignity/.

30. For an excellent discussion of the difference between suicide and death with dignity, see Lonni Shavelson, *A Chosen Death: The Dying Confront Assisted Suicide* (Berkeley: University of California Press, 1995).

31. See Edward Schiappa, *Defining Reality: Definitions and the Politics of Meaning* (Carbondale: Southern Illinois University Press, 2003).

32. See Rebecca Dresser, "Dignity Can Be a Useful Concept in Bioethics," in *Bioethics, Public Moral Argument, and Social Responsibility,* ed. Nancy M. P. King and Michael J. Hyde (New York: Routledge, 2012), 45–54.

33. Marcia Angell, "Marcia Angell: Brittany Maynard Is Changing the Assisted-Dying Debate," November 3, 2014, http://www.dallasnews.com/opinion/latest-columns/20141105-1.ece.

34. Philip Pulleilla and Alex Dobuginskis, "Vatican Official Condemns Maynard Assisted Suicide Case in U.S.," November 4, 2014, http://www.reuters.com/article/2014/11/05/us-usa-assistedsuicide-vatican-idUSKBN0IO1UU20141105.

35. ONTIMETHESHOW, "Brittany Maynard Died—Terminal Cancer Woman Brittany Maynard Ends Her Life [TRIBUTE]," Novermber 2, 2014, https://www.youtube.com/watch?v=gtPhNZgU1jg , Nov 2, 2014.

36. Karoli Kuns, "Brittany Maynard Chose Peaceful Death over Dying from Brain Cancer," November 3, 2014, http://crooksandliars.com/2014/11/brittany-maynard-chose-peaceful-death-over-dying-from-brain-cancer.

37. William Peace, "The Latest Photogenic Face of Assisted Suicide," October 11, 2014, http://badcripple.blogspot.com/2014_10_05_archive.html.

38. During the eighteen months spent reviewing Maynard's story, I never found any media coverage reporting that the first video was not produced by Compassion & Choices. This fact was finally uncovered during a three-hour phone interview with Maynard's husband, Dan Diaz, on April 26, 2016.

39. Raphael Demos, "On Persuasion," *Journal of Philosophy* 29 (1932): 229.

40. See, for example, Ms. Tolisanoi, Period 4 Blog, February 29, 2016, http://tolisanoperiod4.blogspot.com/2016/02/aow-5-brittany-maynard.html; Stuart Chambers, "Legal History Ignored by Opponents of Medically Assisted Death," *Bioethics.Net,* April 29, 2016, http://www.bioethics.net/2016/04/legal-history-ignored-by-opponents-of-medically-assisted-death/; The Brittany Maynard Fund, 2016, http://thebrittanyfund.org/.

41. Maynard, "A New Video for My Friends."

42. Compassion & Choices, "Brittany Maynard Urges Palliative Care Specialist to Stop Misrepresenting Her Case," October 23, 2014, https://www.compassionandchoices.org/2014/10/23/brittany-maynard-urges-palliative-care-specialist-to-stop-misrepresenting-her-case/.

43. Peace, "The Latest Photogenic Face of Assisted Suicide."

44. Ashton Ellis, "Who's Framing Brittany Maynard," October 31, 2014, http://www.thepublicdiscourse.com/2014/10/14020/.

45. Elina Dockterman, "Watch Brittany Maynard's Video in Support of Right-to-Die Legislation," March 25, 2014, http://time.com/3759208/brittany-maynard-right-to-die-video-california/.

46. Political Paula, "Brittany Maynard Is a Hero In Spite of What a Religious, Terminal Cancer Patient Says!," October 23, 2014, https://www.facebook.com/politicalpaula/posts/1562302713985109h; Jim Bouchard, "Death with Dignity: Why Brittany Maynard Is a Hero . . . and So Was My Friend Don," November 3, 2014, http://thinklikeablackbelt.org/2014/11/03/special-post-death-with-dignity-why-brittany-maynard-is-a-heroand-so-was-my-friend-don/; Dileas, "Brittany Maynard Is a Hero," November 5, 2014, http://genxpose.blogspot.com/2014/11/brittany-maynard-is-hero.html; Natasha Lennard, "29-Year-Old Brittany Maynard's Suicide Was Heroic," November 13, 2014, https://news.vice.com/article/29-year-old-brittany-maynards-suicide-was-heroic; Absolute Write, "Death with Dignity Advocate Brittany Maynard Dies in Oregon," November 3, 2014, absolutewrite.com.

47. Emmanuel Levinas, *Time and the Other*, trans. Richard Cohen (Pittsburgh, Pa.: Duquesne University Press, 1987), 73.

48. Emmanuel Levinas, *Otherwise Than Being or Beyond Essence,* trans. Alphonso Lingis (Boston: Klumer, 1991), 144–46.

49. Compassion & Choices, "New Video of Brittany Maynard Released on Her 30th Birthday," November 20, 2014, http://kfor.com/2014/11/20/new-video-of-brittany-maynard-released-on-her-30th-birthday/.

50. Kelly McMann, "Brittany Maynard's Last Words," November 3, 2014, http://q104.cbslocal.com/2014/11/03/brittany-maynards-last-words/.

51. Truth Teller, "Brittany Maynard Was a Coward," November 3, 2014, http://www.topix.com/forum/topstories/TA57OPNL877QHI8KQ.

52. Kara Tippetts, "Dear Brittany: Why We Don't Have to Be So Afraid of Dying and Suffering That We Chose to Die," October 8, 2014, http://www.aholyexperience.com/2014/10/dear-brittany-why-we-dont-have-to-be-so-afraid-of-dying-suffering-that-we-choose-suicide/.

53. Kenneth Burke, *The Rhetoric of Religion: Studies in Logology* (Berkeley: University of California Press, 1970), 33, 272.

54. http://www.theamericanconservative.com/dreher/dont-kill-yourself-brittany-maynard-kara-tippetts/comment-page-1/, October 9, 2014.

55. Steven Ertelt, "Psychologist Questions If Brittany Maynard's Family Pressured Her to Commit Suicide," June 16, 2005, http://www.lifenews.com/2015/06/18/psychologist-wonders-if-brittany-maynards-family-pressured-her-to-commit-suicide/.

56. Jessica Kelly, "Can Christians Support Brittany Maynard's Decision," October 9, 2014, http://jessicakelley.com/2014/10/09/can-christians-support-brittany-maynards-decision/.

57. California governor Jerry Brown signed California's right-to-die bill into law in October 2015.

Chapter 7: Our Posthuman Future

1. President's Council on Bioethics, *Beyond Therapy: Biotechnology and the Pursuit of Happiness* (Washington, D.C.: Regan Books, 2003), 1.

2. Leon Kass, "Ageless Bodies, Happy Souls," *The New Atlantis* 1 (Spring 2003): 9–28, http://www.thenewatlantis.com/publications/ageless-bodies-happy-souls. For background material on bioconservatism, see, for example, Francis Fukuyama, *Our Posthuman Future: Consequences of the Biotechnology Revolution* (New York: Picador, 2002); Ruth Macklin, "The New Conservatives in Bioethics: Who Are They and What Do They Seek?," *Hastings Center Report* 36 (2006): 34–43. Eric Cohen, "Conservative Bioethics and the Search for Wisdom," *Hastings Center Report* 36 (2006): 44–56; Matthew B. Crawford, "Biotechnology and the Modern Liberal Project," *Social Science and Modern Society* 44 (October 2007), 131–36; Tom Koch, *Thieves of Virtue: When Bioethics Stole Medicine* (Cambridge, Mass.: MIT Press, 2012). For discussions that favor a bioconservative perspective on our posthuman future and come from "left-wing" authors, see Bill Joy, "Why the Future Doesn't Need Us," *Wired* 8 (April 2000): 1–2; and Jeremy Rifkin, "Fusion Biopolitics," *Nation,* February 18, 2002, http://www.thenation.com/doc.mhtml?i=20020218&s=rifkin.

3. For a collection of essays that discuss the much-contested issue of the difference between therapy and enhancement, see Julian Savulescu and Nick Bostrum (eds.), *Human Enhancement* (New York: Oxford University Press, 2009).

4. Michael Sandel, *The Case against Perfection: Ethics in the Age of Genetic Engineering* (Cambridge, Mass.: Harvard University Press, 2007), 26–29. Ray Kurzweil's response to this type of thinking is noteworthy: "If we regard a human modified with technology as no longer human, where would we draw the defining line? Is a human with a bionic heart still human? How about someone with a neurological implant? What about two neurological implants? How about someone with 10 nanobots in his brain? How about 500 million nanobots? Should we establish a boundary at 650 million nanobots; under that, you're still human and over that, you're posthuman? Our merger with our technology has aspects of a slippery slope, but one that slides up toward greater promise, not down into Nietzsche's abyss." Ray Kurzweil, *The Singularity Is Near: When Humans Transcend Biology* (New York: Penguin, 2006), 374.

5. Leon Kass, "How Brave a New World?," Catholic Education Resource Center, 2007, http://www.catholiceducation.org/en/science/ethical-issues/how-brave-a-new-world.html.

6. George Annas, Lori Andrews, and Rosario Isasi, "Protecting the Endangered Human: Toward an International Treaty Prohibiting Cloning and Inheritable Alterations," *American Journal of Law and Medicine* 28 (2002): 162. Annas makes a similar argument in his "Genism, Racism, and the Prospect of Genetic Genocide," in *The Future of Values: 21st-Century Talks,* ed. Jerome Binde (New York: United Nations Educational, Scientific and Cultural Organization and Berghahn Books, 2004), 284–88.

7. Allen Buchanan, *Better Than Human: The Promise and Perils of Enhancing Ourselves* (New York: Oxford University Press, 2011), 117.

8. Arthur Caplan, "Roundtable Discussion," in *Neuroethics: Mapping the Field: Conference Proceedings,* ed. Steven J Marcus (San Francisco: Dana Press, 2002), 106.

9. Ronald Bailey, *Liberation Biology: The Scientific and Moral Case for the Biotech Revolution* (New York: Prometheus Books, 2005), 19.

10. Lee Silver, *Challenging Nature: The Clash between Biotechnology and Spirituality* (New York: HarperCollins, 2006), 351.

11. Leon R. Kass, *Life, Liberty, and the Defense of Dignity: The Challenge for Bioethics* (San Francisco: Encounter Books, 2002), 241.

12. See Johann A. R. Roduit, *The Case for Perfection: Ethics in the Age of Human Enhancement* (New York: Peter Lang, 2016). Roduit notes that "bioconservatives themselves rely on a distinct substantive understanding of human perfection while accusing advocates of enhancement of pursuing perfection" (60–61).

13. Bailey, *Liberation Biology,* 246.

14. Ronald Bailey, "Who's Afraid of Posthumanity? A Look at the Growing Left/Right Alliance in Opposition to Biotechnological Progress," in *Biotechnology: Our Future as Human Beings and Citizens,* ed. Sean D. Sutton (Albany: State University of New York Press, 2009), 45.

15. Gregory Stock, *Redesigning Humans: Choosing Our Genes, Changing Our Future* (New York: Mariner Books, 2003), 1–2, 5. On this point, also see James C. Peterson, *Genetic Turning Points: The Ethics of Human Genetic Intervention* (Grand Rapids, Mich.: William B. Eerdmans, 2001).

16. Francis Collins, "The Veritas Forum: The Language of God," http://www.youtube.com/watch?v=DjJAWuzno9Y.

17. Francis S. Collins, *The Language of God* (New York: Free Press, 2006), 20. Further reference to the book will be cited in the text.

18. Abraham Joshua Heschel, *God in Search of Man: A Philosophy of Judaism* (New York: Noonday Press, 1955), 74.

19. Sam Harris, *Moral Landscape: How Science Can Determine Human Values* (New York: Free Press, 2010), 160.

20. Sam Harris, *Letter to a Christian Nation* (New York: Vintage, 2008), vii.

21. Harris, *Letter to a Christian Nation,* ix–xi.

22. Time International, "God vs. Science, Richard Dawkins and Francis Collins" (interviewed by Dan Cray), November 5, 2006, http://inters.org/Dawkins-Collins-Cray-Science.

23. Nick Bostrom, "Why I Want to Be a Posthuman When I Grow Up," in *Medical Enhancement and Posthumanity,* ed. Bert Gordin and Ruth Chadwick (Dordrecht: Springer, 2009), 111–12. For an exceptionally educational discussion of transhumanism, see Bostrum's "The History of Transhumanist Thought," *Journal of Evolution and Technology* 14 (April 2005): 1–25.

24. Nicholas Agar, *Humanity's End: Why We Should Reject Radical Enhancement* (Cambridge, Mass.: MIT Press, 2010), 148.

25. Agar, *Humanity's End,* 11–12, 152, 157–60, 171–72. Also see Michael Hauskeller, *Better Humans?: Understanding the Enhancement Project* (United Kingdom, London: Acumen, 2013).

26. The philosopher, lawyer, literary critic, and transhumanist Russell Blackford takes issue with bioconservatives who assume that "six trite truths about technology" are not appreciated by posthumanists who do not state them explicitly in their writings and public presentations. These truths include (1) "In the real world, technological advances involve compromise and trade-offs"; (2) "Technological advances take place in unexpected ways and find unexpected uses"; (3) "Implanted technologies have disadvantages as well as advantages: e.g., prostheses and implants are often experienced as imperfect and obtrusive, and they wear out"; (4) "Predictions about future technologies and how they will be incorporated into social practice are unreliable"; (5) "Future technologies will sometimes be used for spiteful or malevolent purposes and will typically be used for self-interested ones"; and (6) "Science fiction is one—though certainly not the only—resource available to people, including transhumanists, who want to think about possibilities for our future." Blackford does not defend these six points individually because he "cannot imagine that anyone would disagree with them, once they are stated plainly and concisely. . . . If they are not explicitly stated in transhumanist theories and manifestos, it is most likely because they are considered so obvious that they go without saying, rather than that the authors are unaware of them or disagree with them." See Russell Blackford, "Trite Truths about Technology: A Reply to Ted Peters," in *H+/-: Transhumanism and Its Critics,* ed. Gregory R. Hansell and William Grassie (Philadelphia: Metanexus Institute, 2011), 182–84. Notice that my critical assessment of Bostrum's vision goes beyond the six trite truths that concern Blackford.

27. Heschel, *God in Search of Man,* 75.

28. Cited in B. A. Koenig, H. T. Greely, L. M. McConell, H. L. Silverberg, and T. A. Faffin, "Genetic Testing for BRCA1 and BRCA2: Recommendations of the Stanford Program in Genomics, Ethics, and Society," *Journal of Woman's Health* 7 (1998): 533.

29. For an extensive discussion and literature review on regenerative medicine, see Tristan Keys, Nancy M. P. King, and Anthony Atala, "Faith in Science: Professional and Public Discourse on Regenerative Medicine," in *After the Genome: A Language for Our Biotechnological Future,* eds. Michael J. Hyde and James A. Herrick (Waco, Tex.: Baylor University Press, 2013), 11–40.

30. At the time of this writing, Atala's and his team's most recent project is the lab-grown penis and its transplantation. See, for example, Dara Mohammadi, "The Lab-grown Penis: Approaching a Medical Milestone," *The Guardian,* http://www.theguardian.com/education/2014/oct/04/penis-transplants-anthony-atala-interview. When I talk to my students about lab-grown vaginal organs, they are awestruck. When I talk about lab-grown and transplanted penises, the students typically giggle. Asking the students why their responses were different, I was told that "a penis is funnier." Humor dissipated, however, when I explained that Atala's research is made possible by a $40 million grant from the U.S. military supporting this country's "Wounded Warrior" program. Severe genitalia injuries are not uncommon in war. I added further persuasive context to this fact by quoting Major General Joseph Caravalho Jr. M.D., who is the General of the Armed Forces Institute of Regenerative Medicine (AFIRM) and who had this to say in a personal interview (March 25, 2014) dealing specifically with Atala's research program: "What I think a lot of Americans don't understand is these soldiers and sailors, airmen and Marines, it is just half the battle to have them alive. They will be with us for the next sixty to eighty years, and we are committed to them for that period of time. And it is not simply, you know, when the war is over, it is not a simple matter of saying 'Okay, let's move on?' That person's leg is not coming back. The disfiguring scars on the face are not coming back. So I think the hope is that we continue to offer them a hope for their lives and for their families for the decades to come. . . . This is a great burden that we are placing on [Dr. Atala] and we are relying on him . . . because of this country's sailors, soldiers, airmen, and Marines who have been injured fighting on behalf of the president and this country."

31. John Harris, *Enhancing Evolution: The Ethical Case for Making Better People* (Princeton, N.J.: Princeton University Press, 2007), 3–4.

32. Mary Shelley, *Frankenstein; Or, the Modern Prometheus* (New York: Penguin Books, 1985). Further references to this book will be cited in the text.

33. Marilyn Butler, "Frankenstein and Radical Science," in Mary Shelley, *Frankenstein,* ed. J. Paul Hunter (New York: W. W. Norton, 1996), 307.

34. Michael Kosfield, Marjus Heinricks, Paul J. Zak, Urs Fischbacher, and Ernst Fehr, "Oxytocin Increases Trust in Humans, *Nature* 435 (June 2, 2005): 673–76; also see "DNA Learning Center: Preparing Students and Families to Thrive in the Gene Age," Cold Spring Harbor Laboratory. http://www.dnalc.org/.

35. Carsten K.W. De Dreu, Lindred L. Greer, Michel J. J. Handgraaf, Shaul Shalvi, Gerben A. Van Kleef, Matthijs Baas, Femke S. Ten Velden, Eric Van Dijk, and Sander

W. W. Feith, "The Neuropeptide Oxytocin Regulates Parochial Altruism in Intergroup Conflict among Humans," *Science* 328 (November 6, 2010): 1408–11; Carsten K. W. De Dreu, Lindred L. Greer, Gerben A. Van Kleef, Shaul Shalvi, and Michell J. J. Handgraaf, "Oxytocin Provides Human Ethnocentrism," *Proceedings of the National Academy of Sciences* 108 (2011): 1262–66.

36. The negative effects of moral enhancement are the major reason for arguments cautioning against its promotion. For an excellent review of the literature dealing with the pro and con assessments of moral enhancement, see Jona Specker, Farah Focquaert, Kasper Raus, Sigrid Sterckx, and Maartje Schermer, "The Ethical Desirability of Moral Bioenhancement: A Review of Reasons," *BioMed Central Medical Ethics* 15 (2014): 1–25.

37. Nick Bostrum, "Dignity and Enhancement," in *Human Dignity and Bioethics*, ed. President's Council on Bioethics (Washington, D.C.: President's Council on Bioethics, 2008), 180.

38. Patricia S. Churchland, "Human Dignity from a Neurophilosophical Perspective," in President's Council on Bioethics (ed.), *Human Dignity and Bioethics*, 118.

39. For discussions that relate moral enhancement to cultivating the conditions that favor the good life, see, for example, Elizabeth Fenton, "The Perils of Failing to Enhance: A Reponse to Persson and Savulescu," *Journal of Medical Ethics* 36 (2010): 148–51; Thomas Douglas, "Moral Enhancement," *Journal of Applied Philosophy* 25 (2008): 228–45; David DeGrazia, "Moral Enhancement, Freedom, and What We (Should) Value in Moral Behavior," *Journal of Medical Ethics* 40 (2014): 361–68; James J. Hughes, *Citizen Cyborg: Why Democratic Societies Must Respond to the Redesigned Human of the Future* (Cambridge, Mass.: Westview Press, 2004); James J. Hughes, "Moral Enhancement Requires Multiple Virtues: Toward a Posthuman Model of Character Development," *Cambridge Quarterly of Healthcare Ethics* 24 (January 2015): 86–95.

40. Harris, *Enhancing Evolution;* Ingmar Persson and Julian Savulescu, *Unfit for the Future: The Need for Moral Enhancement* (New York: Oxford University Press, 2012).

41. Persson and Savulescu, *Unfit for the Future*, 9, 121.

42. Heidi Ledford, "CRISPR: The Disruptor," *Nature* 522 (June 2015): 20–24. CRISPR allows scientists to edit genomes with unprecedented precision, efficiency, and flexibility. See also John Harris, *How to Be Good* (New York: Oxford University Press, 2016). Throughout his book, Harris takes issue with various claims made by Persson and Savulescu concerning the necessity and procedures of moral enhancement.

43. Bill McKibben, *Enough: Staying Human in an Engineered Age* (New York: St. Martin's Griffin, 2004), 128.

44. President's Council on Bioethics, *Beyond Therapy*, 27–95. For a much condensed but still quite informative discussion of the PCB's consideration of this and related matters, see Sandel, *The Case against Perfection*, 45–62.

45. Nick Bostrom, "In Defense of Posthuman Dignity," in Hansell and Grassie (eds.), *H±: Transhumanism and Its Critics*, 63.

46. Pierre Teilhard de Chardin, *The Phenomenon of Man*, trans. Bernard Wall (New York: HarperPerennial, 1959), 282–83.

47. Nicholas Agar, *Liberal Eugenics: In Defense of Human Enhancement* (Oxford: Blackwell, 2004), 5.

48. Agar, *Liberal Eugenics,* vii, 5. Agar refines this position in his *Humanity's End.* Also see Franxoise Baylis and Jason Scott Robert, "The Inevitability of Genetic Enhancement Technologies," *Bioethics* 18 (2004): 1–26; Ross Andersen, "Why Cognitive Enhancement Is in Your Future (and Your Past)," *Atlantic* (February 2012), http://www.theatlanticcom/technology/archive/2012/02/why-cognitive-enhancement-is-in-your-future-and-your-past/252566/.

49. Gennady Stolyarov II, *Death Is Wrong* (New York: Rational Argumentor Press/Ria University Press, 2013). Further references to this book will be cited in the text.

50. See Aubrey de Grey and Michael Rae, *Ending Aging: The Rejuvenation Breakthroughs That Could Reverse Human Aging in Our Lifetime* (New York: St. Martin's Griffin, 2008).

51. Mark Walker, "Ship of Fools: Why Transhumanism Is the Best Bet to Prevent the Extinction of Civilization," in Hansell and Grassie (eds.), *H+/-: Transhumansm and Its Critics,* 100.

52. Max More, "True Transhumanism: A Reply to Don Ihde," in Hansell and Grassie (eds.), *H+/-: Transhumanism and Its Critics,* 139.

53. Ted Peters, "Transhumanism and the Posthuman Future: Will Technological Progress Get Us There," in Hansell and Grassie (eds.), *H+/-: Transhumanism and Its Critics,* 173.

54. Hans Moravec, *Robot: Mere Machine to Transcendent Mind* (Oxford: Oxford University Press, 1999); Kurzweil, *The Singularity Is Near: When Humans Transcend Biology.*

55. I mention these three films because I really like them, despite the mixed reviews they received from film critics. I apologize to science fiction film buffs who find my artistic taste lacking in sophistication. I am well aware that there are many more films that speak to the topic of posthumanity. But I am quite comfortable with my choices.

56. *Her,* directed by Spike Jonze, produced by Megan Ellison, Spike Jonze, and Vincent Landay (Los Angeles: Annapuna Pictures, 2013).

57. Joel R. Primack and Nancy Ellen Abrams, *The View from the Center of the Universe* (New York: Riverhead Books, 2006), 234–35.

58. President's Council on Bioethics, *Beyond Therapy,* xvii.

59. Carl Elliott, *Better Than Well: American Medicine Meets the American Dream* (New York: W. W. Norton, 2003), 283.

60. Hayles, *How We Became Posthuman,* 246.

Epilogue

1. Saul D. Alinsky, *Rules for Radicals: A Pragmatic Primer for Realistic Radicals* (New York: Vintage Books, 1971), 3.

2. Plato, *Apology* (40a–b), trans. Hugh Tredennick, in *Collected Dialogues of Plato,* ed. Edith Hamilton and Huntington Cairns (Princeton, N.J.: Princeton University Press, 1961).

3. Collins is critical of Intelligent Design theory (see 181–96), but I do not see how he could dispute my use of the term "design" in the present context.

4. Quoted in Charles H. Kahn, *The Art and Thought of Heraclitus: An Edition of the Fragments with Translation and Commentary* (New York: Cambridge University Press, 1979), 33, Fragment X.

Index